MOSBY'S

OB/Peds & Women's Health
Memory
NoteCards

Visual, Mnemonic, and Memory Aids for Nurses

JoAnn Zerwekh, MSN, EdD, RN

Executive Director
Nursing Education Consultants
Ingram, Texas

CJ Miller
Iowa City, Iowa

Reviewed by

Barbara Pascoe, RN, BA, MA
**Director of Maternity, Gynecology,
 and Pediatrics**
Concord Hospital
Concord, New Hampshire

Deborah A. Terrell, RN, PhD, FNP-BC
Associate Professor
City Colleges of Chicago
Chicago, Illinois

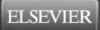

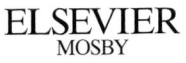

3251 Riverport Lane
St. Louis, Missouri 63043

MOSBY'S OB/PEDS & WOMEN'S HEALTH MEMORY NOTECARDS: ISBN: 978-0-323-08351-5
VISUAL, MNEMONIC, AND MEMORY AIDS FOR NURSES

NOTICES

Knowledge and best practice in this field are constantly changing. As new research and
experience broaden our understanding, changes in research methods, professional prac-
tices, or medical treatment may become necessary. Practitioners and researchers must
always rely on their own experience and knowledge in evaluating and using any information, methods, compounds, or experiments described herein. In using such information
or methods they should be mindful of their own safety and the safety of others, including
parties for whom they have a professional responsibility.

With respect to any drug or pharmaceutical products identified, readers are advised to
check the most current information provided (i) on procedures featured or (ii) by the manu-
facturer of each product to be administered, to verify the recommended dose or formula,
the method and duration of administration, and contraindications. It is the responsibility of
the practitioners, relying on their own experience and knowledge of their patients, to make
diagnoses, to determine dosages and the best treatment for each individual patient, and
to take all appropriate safety precautions.

To the fullest extent of the law, neither the Publisher nor the authors, contributors, or edi-
tors, assume any liability for any injury and/or damage to persons or property as a matter
of products liability, negligence or otherwise, or from any use or operation of any methods,
products, instructions, or ideas contained in the material herein.

International Standard Book Number: 978-0-323-08351-5

Executive Editor: Kristin Geen
Development Editor: Lauren Harms
Publishing Services Manager: Jeff Patterson
Project Manager: Megan Isenberg
Designer: Ashley Eberts
Cover Art: CJ Miller

Printed in China

Last digit is the print number: 9 8 7 6 5 4

Working together to grow
libraries in developing countries

www.elsevier.com | www.bookaid.org | www.sabre.org

ELSEVIER   BOOK AID International   Sabre Foundation

Contents

PEDIATRICS

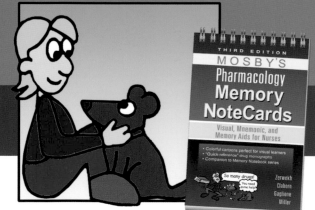

FINALLY, OB/PEDS AND WOMEN'S HEALTH MADE CLEAR!
USE YOUR NOTECARDS AS A:

- Companion study guide for obstetrics, pediatrics, and women's health texts
- Quick review for examinations
- Reference to use with other health care texts

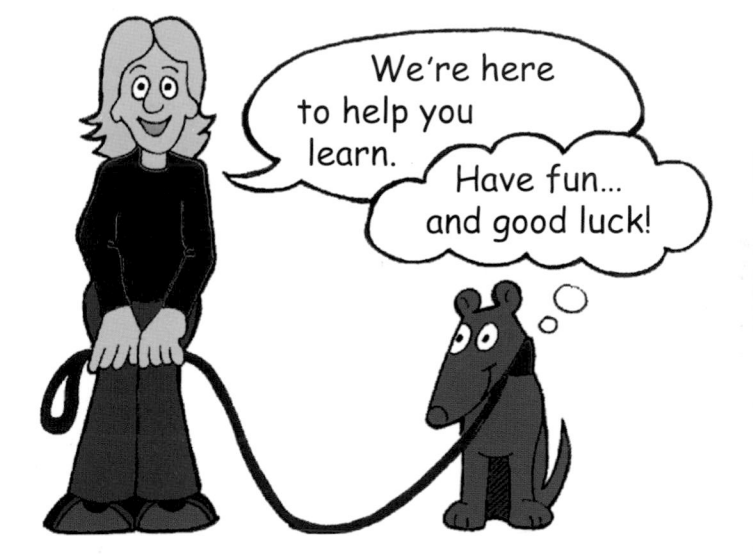

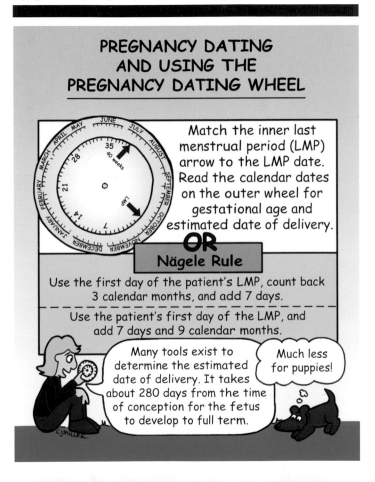

Pregnancy Dating and Using the Pregnancy Dating Wheel

DEFINITION

- EDD is the patient's *estimated date of delivery*.
- EDB is a newer term and refers to the *estimated date of birth*.
- Gestational age of the fetus can be determined after the EDD and refers to the age of the fetus in weeks and days.
- Many tools are used to determine the patient's EDD.

NÄGELE RULE

- Using the first day of the patient's last menstrual period (LMP), count back 3 calendar months and add 7 days, or use the patient's first day of the patient's LMP and add 9 calendar months and 7 days.
- Example: LMP is 3/10/2012 and EDD is 12/17/2012.
- Most patients deliver within 7 days of their EDDs or EDBs.

TRANSVAGINAL ULTRASOUND

- Transvaginal ultrasound is used between 4 and 10 weeks and is the most accurate form of pregnancy dating.

NURSING IMPLICATIONS

1. If a pregnancy dating wheel is used, match the inner LMP arrow to the LMP date. Read the calendar dates on the outer wheel for the EDD.
2. Teach the patient that the EDD or EDB is an estimate and that most patients deliver within 7 days of the projected date.

Serious/life-threatening implications	Important nursing implications
Common clinical findings	Patient teaching

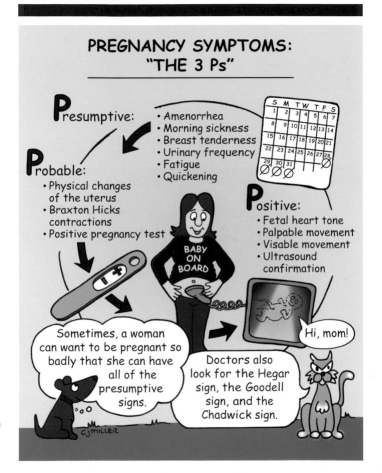

Pregnancy Symptoms: "The 3 Ps"

DEFINITION

The presumptive and probable signs of pregnancy are those felt by the mother and seen by the physician. These signs and symptoms do not diagnose a pregnancy because they can be attributed to other conditions of the female reproductive system. The positive signs of pregnancy are those that confirm the pregnancy.

SIGNS AND SYMPTOMS

- Presumptive signs of pregnancy are the least reliable predictors of pregnancy.
  - Amenorrhea
  - Nausea and vomiting ("morning sickness")
  - Breast changes (e.g., deeper pigmentation of the areola)
  - Urinary frequency
  - Fatigue
  - Quickening (feeling fetal movement; occurs around 16 to 20 weeks)
  - Striae gravidarum, chloasma ("mask of pregnancy"), linea nigra (vertical pigmented line on abdomen)
- Probable signs of pregnancy include:
  - Hegar sign—softening of lower uterine segment
  - Chadwick sign—bluish discoloration of vagina
  - Goodell sign—softening of cervical lip
  - Positive pregnancy test, urine or serum
  - Abdominal enlargement
  - Braxton Hicks contractions
- Positive signs of pregnancy include:
  - Visualization of the fetus using ultrasound
  - Auscultation of the fetal heart rate by Doppler as early as the 6th week of gestation; reliable at the 8th and 9th weeks; by fetal stethoscope between the 16th and 20th weeks
  - Visualization or palpation of fetal movement by a health care practitioner

Serious/life-threatening implications	Important nursing implications
Common clinical findings	Patient teaching

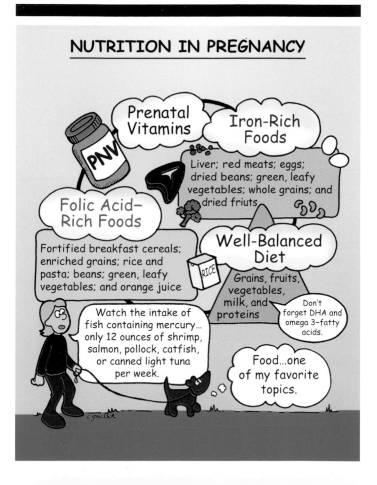

Nutrition in Pregnancy

DEFINITION

A healthful diet before conception and throughout pregnancy is important to ensure adequate nutrients for the growing fetus.

RISK FACTORS

- Adolescent pregnancy
- Bizarre or faddish food habits
- Abuse of nicotine, alcohol, or drugs
- Low or high weight for height of mother and frequent pregnancies
- Low hemoglobin and hematocrit levels

KEY POINTS

- Total maternal weight gain and pattern of weight gain are important.
  - First trimester (singleton pregnancy): 1 to 2.5 kg total weight gain
  - Second and third trimesters (singleton pregnancy): 0.4 kg per week for a normal weight woman, 0.3 kg per week for an overweight woman, and 0.5 kg per week for an underweight woman
  - First trimester (twins): 0.3 to 0.8 kg per week
  - Second trimester (twins): 0.45 kg per week
  - Third trimester (twins): 0.3 to 0.6 kg per week
  - Weight gain of more than 3 kg in a month after the 20th week often indicates the development of preeclampsia.
- Women with normal body mass index (BMI) should gain between 11.5 and 16 kg during pregnancy.
  - Underweight women should gain between 12.5 and 18 kg during pregnancy.
  - Overweight women should gain between 7 and 11.5 kg during pregnancy.
  - Obese women should gain at least 7 kg.

NURSING IMPLICATIONS

1. Encourage a diet with iron-rich foods and foods high in folic acid.
2. Explain the importance of prenatal vitamins.
3. Monitor weight gain as calculated by using the mother's BMI.
4. Teach the mother the importance of an adequate diet before, during, and after pregnancy.
5. Teach the mother how to individualize her diet to achieve adequate nutritional intake.
6. Monitor for nutrition-related discomforts of pregnancy—nausea, vomiting, constipation, and pyrosis (heartburn).

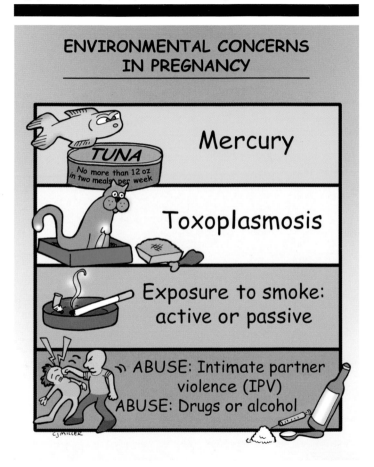

Environmental Concerns in Pregnancy

LEAD PAINT–CONTAMINATED WATER

- Lead exposure can lead to delays in physical and mental development, lower IQ levels, shortened attention spans, and increased behavioral problems.
- Nursing management: Teach pregnant women to have their water supply tested and to use bottled water if their water has high levels of lead.

TOXOPLASMOSIS

- *Toxoplasma gondii* is transmitted by cat feces, contaminated soil, or infected meat that is raw or undercooked.
- Parasite is spread transplacentally if the mother acquires infection.
- Neonatal effects: Low birth weight, enlarged spleen, jaundice, coagulation disorders, blindness, deafness, seizures, hydrocephalus, microcephaly
- Nursing management: Teach the mother to cook meat thoroughly, avoid uncooked eggs and unpasteurized milk, wash fruits and vegetables before consuming, and avoid contact with cat litter boxes, sandboxes, and garden soil.

MERCURY

- Shark, swordfish, marlin, king mackerel, albacore or white tuna, and tilefish have high levels of mercury.
- Shrimp, canned or light tuna, salmon, pollack, and catfish have smaller amounts of mercury.
- Nursing management: Teach pregnant women to avoid fish high in mercury content and limit intake to no more than 12 oz (in two meals) per week.

EXPOSURE TO SMOKE

- A causal relation exists between maternal smoking and reduced birth weight.
- Smoking causes a decrease in placental perfusion.
- Nursing management: Encourage pregnant women to stop smoking and to avoid areas where exposure to secondary smoke can occur.

ABUSE

- Intimate partner violence occurs from either a current or former intimate partner and can be physical, sexual, or emotional abuse, as well as threats of abuse.
  - Nursing management: Teach pregnant women to recognize the signs of IPV and to develop a personal safety plan.
- Alcohol or drugs
  - Alcohol can cause fetal alcohol syndrome, fetal alcohol effects, learning disabilities, and hyperactivity.
  - Drugs can have teratogenic effects and cause metabolic disturbances and withdrawal in the neonate.

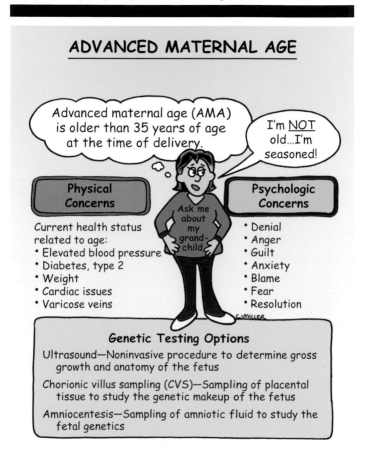

Advanced Maternal Age

DEFINITION

Advanced maternal age (AMA) is usually considered over 35 years of age at the time of delivery.

Women older than 35 years may be less fertile than younger women because they tend to ovulate (release an egg from the ovaries) less frequently.

RISK FACTORS

- Common factors that interfere with conception include:
  - Endometriosis
  - Blocked fallopian tubes
  - Fibroids
- Down syndrome in infants of AMA mothers is the most common chromosomal birth defect.

SIGNS AND SYMPTOMS

- Physical concerns
  - Hypertension, obesity, type 2 diabetes, varicose veins, and other chronic conditions
- Psychologic concerns
  - Denial, anger, guilt, anxiety, and fear

NURSING IMPLICATIONS

1. Provide routine prenatal care and monitor for age-related pregnancy conditions (e.g., type 2 diabetes, hypertension, obesity).
2. Discuss genetic counseling.
3. Promote discussions of changing and reordering life priorities as a result of the pregnancy.
4. Teach the importance of early prenatal care and reportable signs during pregnancy.

Serious/life-threatening implications   Important nursing implications

Common clinical findings   Patient teaching

POSTPARTUM DEPRESSION

- Strong feelings of sadness
- Crying for no reason
- Feeling unable to care for self or for others
- Loss of appetite
- Loss of interest in appearance
- Inability to fall asleep, waking up early, or sleeping too much
- Difficulty concentrating
- Decreased interest in activities
- Feelings of worthlessness
- Thoughts of harming self or others

I am just so sad...I don't want to hold my baby... I just don't care.

Nursing Actions
- Assess safety issues.
- Assess medication use.
- Observe changes in behaviors and moods.
- Refer to appropriate medical specialties.

Postpartum Depression

DEFINITION

Almost 70% of women experience a mild depression ("baby blues") after delivery; however, their functioning is not impaired. Others experience a more serious depression that affects the interaction of mothers and infants.

RISK FACTORS

- Prenatal depression, low self-esteem, stress, and a lack of social support
- Marital or relationship problems, "difficult" infant temperament, and unplanned or unwanted pregnancy

SIGNS AND SYMPTOMS

- Postpartum blues (baby blues): Begin during the first week after delivery and last a couple of days to 2 weeks. Signs and symptoms include insomnia, fatigue, tearfulness, and anxiety.
- Postpartum depression: Signs include irritability, feelings of guilt about having depressive feelings, rejection of the infant (often caused by abnormal jealousy), odd food cravings (sweet desserts), binges, abnormal appetite, and weight gain.
- Postpartum psychosis: Is a rare condition. Signs include confusion, agitation, bizarre behavior, hallucinations, delusions, and depression or euphoria.

MEDICAL MANAGEMENT

- Postpartum depression: Psychotherapy and medications (selective serotonin reuptake inhibitors [SSRIs], tricyclic antidepressants)
- Postpartum psychosis: Hospitalization and antidepressant and antipsychotic medications

NURSING IMPLICATIONS

1. Support the mother during postpartum blues, and reassure her that it is self-limiting; refer her to a psychiatric care provider if symptoms do not subside in 2 weeks.
2. Demonstrate a caring attitude, and encourage her to talk about her feelings.
3. Provide anticipatory guidance (e.g., need for adequate rest and nutrition).
4. Promote enhanced sensitivity to infant cues.
5. Teach about "kangaroo" (skin-to-skin) care to promote bonding.

Serious/life-threatening implications   Important nursing implications

Common clinical findings   Patient teaching

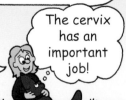

Incompetent Cervix

DEFINITION

Incompetent cervix is also known as cervical insufficiency or recurrent premature dilation of the cervix. This condition usually occurs in the second trimester of pregnancy. The woman is able to become pregnant but cannot bring the pregnancy to term.

RISK FACTORS

- Cervical trauma from childbirth, multiple dilation and curettage (D&C) procedures, and recurrent therapeutic abortions
- Congenital short cervix, cervical biopsy, and cervical abnormalities

SIGNS AND SYMPTOMS

- Passive and painless dilation of the cervix

MEDICAL MANAGEMENT

- Diagnosis: Ultrasound to measure cervical length (Less than 25 mm is considered a short cervix.)
  - Maternal history of repeated pregnancy losses at early gestational age
- Medical treatment: Bedrest, hydration, and tocolysis
- Surgical treatment: Cervical cerclage
  - Risks of cervical cerclage: Rupture of membranes (ROM), preterm labor (PTL), and infection

NURSING IMPLICATIONS

1. Nursing care after cerclage
   - Monitor the patient for contractions, bleeding, ROM, and signs of infection such as fever, uterine tenderness, or foul-smelling discharge.
   - Provide emotional support and use therapeutic communication in dealing with the patient's emotional response to the pregnancy and procedure.
2. Patient teaching
   - Rest. Avoid heavy lifting or prolonged standing; refrain from intercourse; take tocolytic medications as ordered; force fluids; and observe and report any signs of infection, contractions, or ROM.
   - The patient should proceed to the hospital or call 9-1-1 if she feels perineal pressure or the urge to push.
3. Follow-up care
   - Serial ultrasounds determine cervical length.
   - The cerclage is usually removed around the 37th week or may be left in place for future pregnancies; delivery is then performed by cesarean section.

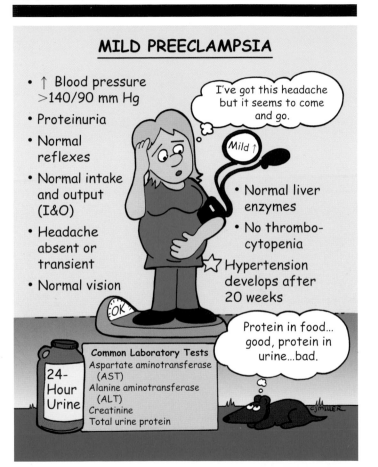

Mild Preeclampsia

DEFINITION

Preeclampsia is a multisystem syndrome specific to pregnancy. Preeclampsia is complicated by reduced organ perfusion related to systemic vasospasm. Symptoms appear after 20 weeks and range from mild to severe.

SIGNS AND SYMPTOMS

- Cardinal signs: Hypertension and proteinuria
- Blood pressure (BP): 140/90 mm Hg taken two times, 4 to 6 hours apart
- Transient headache (HA) and transient irritability
- Fetal effects: May include decreased placental profusion leading to intra-uterine growth restriction and fetal intolerance to labor in the form of late decelerations.

LABORATORY FINDINGS

- Proteinuria ≥1+ on urine dipstick or >0.3 g in a 24-hour urine specimen

MEDICAL MANAGEMENT

- May be taken care of at home if the BP is stable and the patient remains complaint free.
- Bedrest with limited activity will improve uteroplacental profusion.
- Maternal surveillance: Includes daily BP readings, weight, and possibly urine protein.
- Fetal surveillance: Includes biweekly nonstress tests (NSTs), serial ultrasounds for growth, daily fetal movement counting, and biophysical profiles as ordered.

NURSING IMPLICATIONS

- Patient compliance with the plan of care is necessary for success.
- Bedrest may cause muscle atrophy, a decrease in cardiovascular endurance, and severe boredom.
- Teach physical therapy techniques to combat prolonged bedrest.
- Help the patient find pleasing diversional activities to combat boredom.
- Instruct the patient in the proper use of BP equipment, daily weights, and the urine dipstick.
- Instruct the patient in daily movement counting.
- Teach patient the signs and symptoms of worsening preeclampsia and the need to report these symptoms immediately to the physician.
- Reinforce the need for the patient's compliance with at-home instructions and the need to keep all appointments.

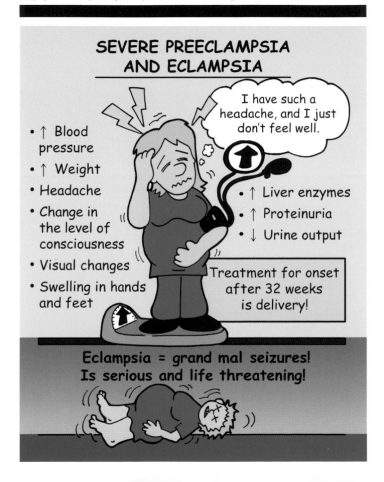

Severe Preeclampsia and Eclampsia

DEFINITION

Severe preeclampsia is a multisystem syndrome specific to pregnancy.
Eclampsia is seizure activity in a patient diagnosed with preeclampsia.

SIGNS AND SYMPTOMS OF SEVERE PREECLAMPSIA

- Cardinal signs: Hypertension and proteinuria
- Blood pressure (BP): >160/110 mm Hg on two separate occasions
- Headaches (HAs), confusion, blurred vision, severe irritability, pulmonary edema, and epigastric, or right upper quadrant (RUQ) pain
- Nausea and vomiting, edema of the hands and face, weight gain, hyper-reflexia >3+, urinary output of <30 ml/hr, and general malaise
- Decreased placental profusion leading to intrauterine growth restriction, fetal intolerance to labor in the form of late decelerations, and fetal demise

LABORATORY FINDINGS

- Proteinuria >2+, 3+ on urine dipstick, or >2 g in 24-hour urine specimen
- Aspartate aminotransferase (AST) >50 U/L and alanine aminotransferase (ALT) >50 U/L, creatinine >1.32 mg/dl, and lactic acid dehydrogenase (LDH) >600 U/L

MEDICAL MANAGEMENT

- Deliver neonate.
- Administer an anticonvulsant (magnesium sulfate) to prevent seizures.
- Administer an antihypertensive medication (e.g., hydralazine, labetalol)
- Administer corticosteroids for fetal lung maturity if the patient is less than 34 weeks' gestation. Restrict fluid intake to 125 ml/hr.
- Conduct serial laboratory values to assess for HELLP syndrome.

NURSING IMPLICATIONS

- Focused assessment should include questions regarding HAs, blurred vision, and the presence of epigastric pain.
- Focused assessments include loss of consciousness (LOC), BP, pulse (P), respiration rate (RR), lung sounds, pulse oximetry, generalized edema, hourly intake and output with urine dipstick for protein and specific gravity, deep-tendon reflexes (DTRs), and daily weights at the same time each day.
- Provide a quiet environment. Room should be closed to staff. Seizure precautions should be in place. Emergency equipment should be readily available and in working condition.
- Magnesium should be continued 24 to 48 hours after delivery; check levels.
- Report any worsening symptoms, especially HAs.

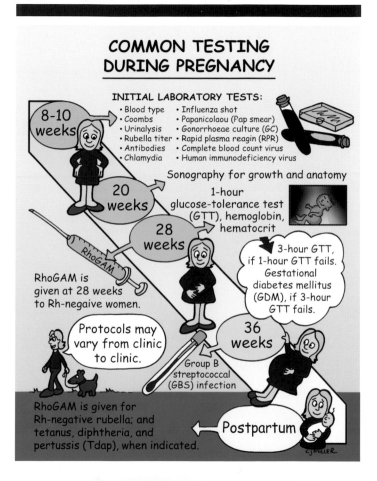

Common Testing during Pregnancy

- **Initial tests** are performed at the first prenatal visit, usually at 8 to 10 weeks:
  - Complete blood count (CBC) to detect anemia or infections
    - African-American: Hemoglobin electrophoresis to detect sickle cell anemia
  - Blood type and Rh factor for irregular antibodies (e.g., anti D)
    - Indirect Coombs test for patients who are Rh-negative to screen for possible Rh incompatibility between the patient and fetus
  - Rubella titer
  - Human immunodeficiency virus (HIV) and hepatitis B testing
  - Tuberculosis (TB) skin test for those patients at risk (e.g., immigrants)
  - Urinalysis and culture and sensitivity (UA/C&S) testing to rule out urinary tract infections and hematuria
  - Papanicolaou (Pap) smear to screen for cervical cancer
  - Vaginal and rectal cultures to screen for gonorrhea, chlamydia, human papilloma virus, and herpes genitalis
  - Venereal disease research laboratory (VDRL) or rapid plasma regain (RPR) testing to screen for syphilis
  - Ultrasound to confirm pregnancy and establish the patient's estimated date of delivery (EDD)
- **16 to 18 weeks**
  - Triple or quad screen to detect Down syndrome and neural tube defects
- **20 weeks**
  - Ultrasound to determine fetal growth, placental location, and amniotic fluid volume (AFV)
- **24 to 28 weeks**
  - 1-hour glucose screen <140 mg/dl to test for gestational diabetes
  - If the test is abnormal, the 3-hour glucose screen is performed. If any two out of the four results are abnormal, the patient is said to have gestational diabetes mellitus (GDM).
    - Nursing care for 3-hour screen includes nothing by mouth (NPO) for 12 hours, no smoking, and no caffeine.
- **28 weeks**
  - Repeat Coombs test, and give the first dose of RhoGAM to patients who are Rh-negative.
- **36 weeks**
  - Perform perineal and rectal swabs for *group B streptococcal infection* (GBS).
- Ultrasound of the fetus can be performed at any time to determine fetal well-being, AFV, and placenta function.

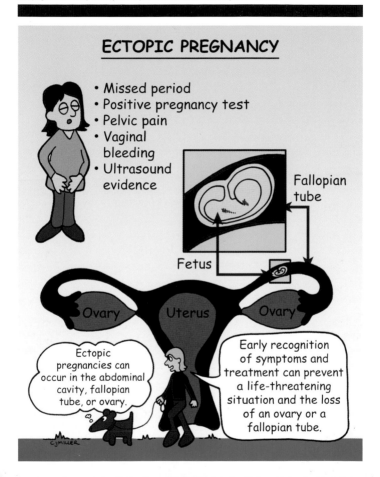

Ectopic Pregnancy

DEFINITION

Ectopic pregnancy is any pregnancy outside of the uterus. Ectopic pregnancy usually occurs in the outer one third of the fallopian tube.

RISK FACTORS

- Pelvic inflammatory disease (PID), infertility, tubal ligation, reversal of tubal ligation, and smoking
- Use of an intrauterine device (IUD), low progesterone levels, multiple elective abortions, and previous ectopic pregnancy

SIGNS AND SYMPTOMS

- Before rupture of the tube: Missed menstrual period; abdominal pain, tenderness, and fullness; and dark-red vaginal bleeding
- After rupture of the tube: Abdominal pain, syncope, shoulder pain, shock out of proportion to the noted blood loss, and Cullen sign (periumbilical darkening of the skin caused by intraperitoneal hemorrhage)

MEDICAL MANAGEMENT

- Testing
  - Blood work for beta–human chorionic gonadotropin (β-hCG) and progesterone levels
  - Transvaginal ultrasound to confirm intrauterine or tubal pregnancy
- Can be nonsurgical or surgical

NURSING IMPLICATIONS

1. Assess abdomen for pain type, location, intensity, and amount and type of vaginal bleeding.
2. Monitor vital signs, menstrual pad count, and syncope.
3. Insert intravenous (IV) large-bore needle, and administer normal saline.
4. Obtain laboratory work: Complete blood count (CBC), blood type, and Rh status.
5. Control pain.
6. Prepare patient for surgery.
7. Postoperatively, administer RhoGAM to the patient who is Rh negative, and begin grief counseling.

Serious/life-threatening implications	Important nursing implications
Common clinical findings	Patient teaching

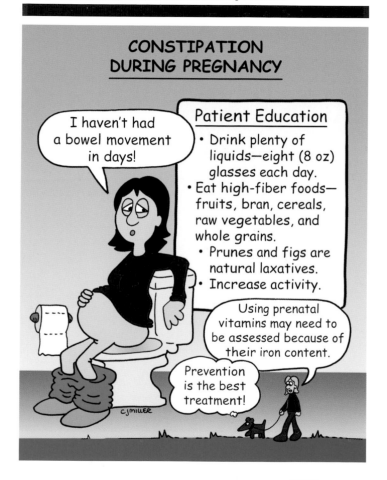

Constipation during Pregnancy

DEFINITION

Constipation is a common problem during pregnancy and occurs as a result of slowed gastrointestinal tract motility because of the effects of progesterone, which increases the resorption of water and a drying of the stool. The problem may be compounded later in pregnancy by the pressure of the growing uterus on the rectum. Iron supplements, particularly in high doses, can make constipation worse.

RISK FACTORS

- Growing uterus
- Iron supplements
- Low-fiber diet

SIGNS AND SYMPTOMS

- Passage of a hard, dry stool
- Abdominal pain or discomfort
- Difficult and infrequent bowel movements

NURSING IMPLICATIONS

1. Promote improved bowel function by increasing the intake of fiber (e.g., brain, whole grains, popcorn, raw or lightly cooked vegetables), which helps create a bulky stool to stimulate peristalsis.
2. Encourage adequate fluid intake (50 ml/kg/day, approximately 8 to 10 glasses) to hydrate the fiber and increase the bulk of the stool.
3. Encourage physical activity—walking, swimming, water aerobics—to stimulate bowel motility.
4. Teach the patient that over-the-counter laxative pills and enemas are not recommended for the treatment of constipation during pregnancy because they may stimulate uterine contractions and cause dehydration.
5. Teach the patient that mineral oils should not be used during pregnancy because an increased reduction in nutrient absorption will occur.

Serious/life-threatening implications   Important nursing implications

Common clinical findings   Patient teaching

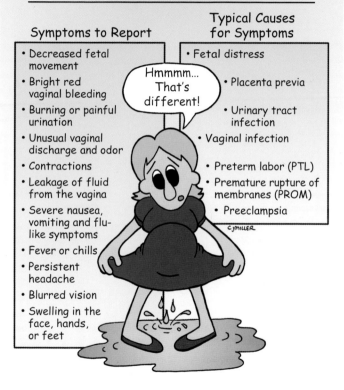

Patient Reportable Symptoms during Pregnancy

DEFINITION

The following is a list of signs and symptoms (S&S) that must be reported to the patient's health care provider and what they typically indicate. The nurse's responsibility is to educate the patient on these S&S. The nurse must also be aware of each S&S and its possible effect on the pregnancy.

REPORTABLE SIGNS AND SYMPTOMS

- Bleeding: Miscarriage, ectopic pregnancy, placenta previa, and abruptio placenta
- Persistent and severe nausea and vomiting: Hyperemesis gravidarum
- Burning or painful urination with or without flank pain: Urinary tract infection (UTI), obstructed ureter, renal calculi, and pyelonephritis
- Fever and chills: Infection
- Diarrhea: Infection
- Persistent headache (HA) not relieved by acetaminophen: Hypertension or preeclampsia
- Visual disturbances such as blurred vision, double vision, or scotoma: Preeclampsia
- Epigastric pain not relieved by antacid: Preeclampsia, HELLP (hemolysis, elevated liver enzymes, low platelet count) syndrome
- Swelling of hands and face: Preeclampsia
- Leakage of fluid or sudden discharge before 37 weeks: Preterm premature rupture of membranes
- Contractions, pelvic pressure, cramping, backache, or increase in vaginal discharge before 37 weeks: Preterm labor
- Change in fetal movement, either decreased or absent: Fetal compromise or fetal death

Serious/life-threatening implications	Important nursing implications
Common clinical findings	Patient teaching

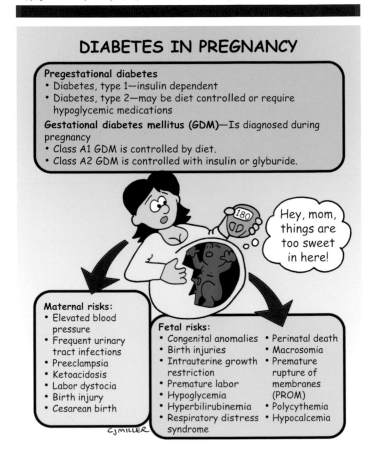

Diabetes in Pregnancy

DEFINITION

- Pregestational diabetes is diagnosed before pregnancy. Pregestational diabetes is type 1 or type 2.
- Gestational diabetes mellitus (GDM) is any degree of glucose intolerance diagnosed during pregnancy.
- Class A1 GDM is controlled by diet and exercise.
- Class A2 GDM is controlled with insulin or glyburide.

RISK FACTORS FOR GDM

- Older than 30 years of age, family history of type 2 diabetes, history of newborn weighing less than 9 pounds, or polyhydramnios
- Unexplained stillbirth, miscarriage, or infant born with congenital anomalies
- Increased blood pressure, recurrent infections

DIAGNOSIS FOR GDM

- One-hour glucose screen at 24 to 28 weeks; should be <140 mg/dl.
- For a blood glucose >140 mg/dl, a 3-hour oral glucose tolerance test (OGTT) is performed. The patient is positive for GDM if two or more blood levels are elevated during the screen.

COMPLICATIONS OF GDM

- Maternal complications: Early pregnancy loss, shoulder dystocia, cesarean birth, labor dystocias, operative vaginal birth, polyhydramnios, infections, hypoglycemia, ketoacidosis, and hypertension
- Fetal complications: Congenital anomalies or macrosomia in the pregestational diabetic, sudden unexplained stillbirth, injuries as a result of delivery dystocias, respiratory distress syndrome (RDS), polycythemia, hyperbilirubinemia, and hypoglycemia after birth

NURSING IMPLICATIONS

1. Monitor glucose level, diet, and exercise during the antepartum period.
2. To ensure patient safety, provide glucose and continuous fetal monitoring and watch for signs of slow labor or inadequate fetal descent during labor. Be prepared for emergency cesarean birth.
3. Monitor for glucose control, possible infections, postpartum hemorrhage, preeclampsia, and problems with breast-feeding in the postpartum period.
4. Monitor newborn for hypoglycemia, especially in the first 24 hours.
5. Teach glucose monitoring, diet, exercise, fetal movement counting, and the signs and symptoms of both hypoglycemia and hyperglycemia.

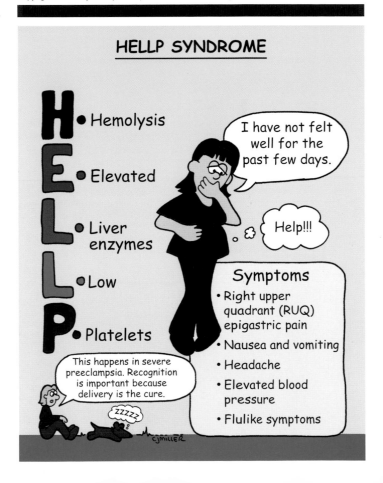

HELLP Syndrome

DEFINITION

HELLP syndrome is usually associated with severe preeclampsia and is the laboratory diagnosis of **H**emolysis, **E**levated **L**iver enzymes, and **L**ow **P**latelets. Patients may have HELLP syndrome without hypertension and proteinuria.
- Fetal implications: Hypoxia, related to uteroplacental insufficiency

RISK FACTORS

- Preeclampsia
- Older Caucasian, multiparous mother

SIGNS AND SYMPTOMS

- Flulike symptoms or general malaise and epigastric or RUQ pain
- Nausea, vomiting, headache, jaundice, and hematuria

MEDICAL MANAGEMENT

- Laboratory tests: Complete blood count (CBC) with platelet count, aspartate aminotransferase (AST), alanine aminotransferase (ALT), lactic acid dehydrogenase (LDH), prothrombin time (PT), partial prothrombin time (PTT), fibrinogen, fibrin split products (FSP), and electrolytes
  - Results: Platelets <100,000; AST >72 U/L; ALT >50 U/L; LDH >600 U/L; abnormal peripheral blood smear with schistocytes or burr cells present
  - Clotting studies usually remain normal.
- Fetal testing: Nonstress test (NST), biophysical profile (BPP), weight, amniocentesis for fetal lung maturity, corticosteroid therapy for the fetus <34 weeks gestational age
  - Continuous electronic fetal monitoring (EFM) during labor with close observation for late decelerations

NURSING IMPLICATIONS

1. Obtain head-to-toe assessments, including focused assessments on the CNS, cardiovascular system, lungs, liver, and kidneys.
2. Implement monitoring for preeclampsia or severe preeclampsia.
3. Monitor for complications of renal failure, pulmonary edema, ruptured liver hematoma, disseminated intravascular clotting (DIC), placental abruption, and preterm birth.
4. Prevent eclampsia, treat hypertension, and correct coagulopathy.
5. Be prepared for emergency delivery, and continue to monitor postpartum for 48 hours.

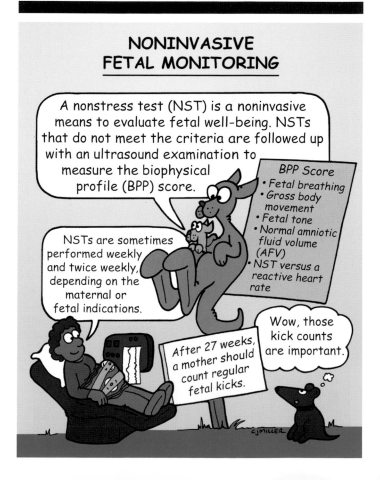

Noninvasive Fetal Monitoring

KICK COUNTS

- The mother assesses fetal movement by counting kicks.
- Various protocols are available for counting fetal kicks:
  - Count for 30 minutes three times each day.
  - Count for 1 hour; if fewer than 10 movements are felt, continue counting another hour; if still fewer than 10 movements are felt after 2 hours, notify the health care provider.
- Teach the mother the importance of this easy, convenient method of evaluating the condition of the fetus on a daily basis.

NONSTRESS TEST

- Evaluates the ability of the fetal heart to accelerate; is often associated with movement.
- The mother is usually seated in a recliner chair or placed in side-lying position with an external electronic fetal monitor used to detect fetal heart rate (FHR), any contractions, and fetal movement.
- Results are noted as reactive (reassuring) and nonreactive (nonreassuring).
  - Reactive: Two FHR accelerations with or without fetal movement occurring within 20 minutes and peaking at least 15 beats per minute above the baseline and lasting 15 seconds (15×15) from baseline to baseline. Acoustic stimulation with a vibroacoustic stimulator of 1 second that elicits similar FHR accelerations is also reassuring.
  - Nonreactive: Tracing does not demonstrate required characteristics of a reactive tracing within 40 minutes.

BIOPHYSICAL PROFILE (BPP)

- Assesses five parameters: (1) nonstress test, (2) fetal breathing movements, (3) gross fetal movements, (4) fetal tone, and (5) amniotic fluid volume (AFV). The last four parameters require ultrasound.
- If ultrasound parameters are reassuring, then the nonstress test is not essential.
- Scoring is based on 10 points with 8 to 10 points considered as normal or reassuring; 6 points as equivocal; and less than 4 points as abnormal or nonreassuring; delivery may be considered.

Serious/life-threatening implications	Important nursing implications
Common clinical findings	Patient teaching

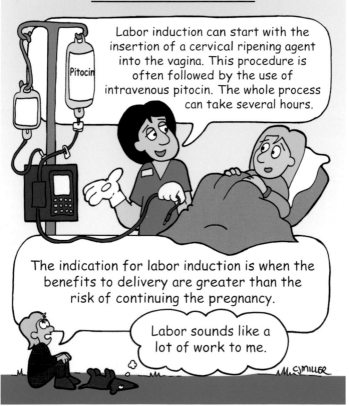

Labor Induction

DEFINITION

Types of labor induction include amniotomy because rupturing the membranes stimulates uterine contractions if the cervix is favorable. Cervical ripening with prostaglandin E2 or misoprostol (Cytotec) or intravenous (IV) oxytocin (Pitocin) may be given to stimulate contractions. Intracervical inserts, which are hydrophilic (moisture attracting), may be used to stretch and soften the cervix.

RISKS

- Uterine hyperstimulation, uterine rupture, maternal water intoxication caused by Pitocin's antidiuretic effects

BISHOP SCORE

- Uses five factors to estimate cervical readiness: (1) cervical dilation, (2) effacement, (3) consistency, (4) position, and (5) fetal station.
- Scoring is based on 10; the higher the score, the greater likelihood of success; a score of 7 in a primipara is favorable.

NURSING IMPLICATIONS

1. Monitor fetal heart rate throughout cervical ripening.
2. Note the administration procedure and precautions for prostaglandin gels, vaginal inserts (Cervidil), and Cytotec.
3. Pitocin needs careful monitoring because it is administered via a piggyback IV with both IVs on an infusion pump; therefore the Pitocin can be stopped if complications develop.
   - Fetal monitoring should be in place.
   - Pitocin is started slowly and increased gradually.
   - Assess maternal vital signs before increasing oxytocin infusion rate.
   - Discontinue IV oxytocin and turn on the primary IV solution if any of the following occur:
     - Nonreassuring fetal heart rate pattern; absent variability; abnormal baseline rate
     - Sustained uterine contractions lasting longer than 90 seconds
     - Insufficient relaxation of the uterus between contractions
     - Contractions occurring more often than every 2 minutes
     - Repeated late decelerations or prolonged decelerations

Serious/life-threatening implications	Important nursing implications
Common clinical findings	Patient teaching

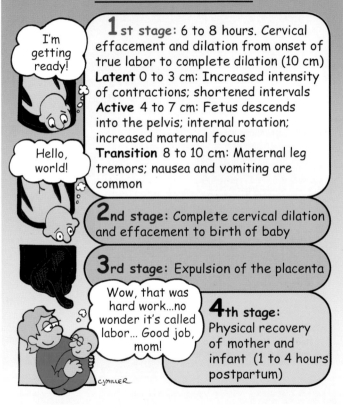

STAGES OF LABOR

1st stage: 6 to 8 hours. Cervical effacement and dilation from onset of true labor to complete dilation (10 cm)
Latent 0 to 3 cm: Increased intensity of contractions; shortened intervals
Active 4 to 7 cm: Fetus descends into the pelvis; internal rotation; increased maternal focus
Transition 8 to 10 cm: Maternal leg tremors; nausea and vomiting are common

2nd stage: Complete cervical dilation and effacement to birth of baby

3rd stage: Expulsion of the placenta

4th stage: Physical recovery of mother and infant (1 to 4 hours postpartum)

I'm getting ready!

Hello, world!

Wow, that was hard work...no wonder it's called labor... Good job, mom!

CJMILLER

Stages of Labor

FIRST STAGE OF LABOR—LATENT PHASE

- Lasts approximately 6 to 8 hours but could be longer for primipara.
- Contractions are mild to moderate and 5 to 30 minutes apart; each contraction lasts for 30 to 45 seconds.
- Encourage comfort measures such as walking. Provide explanations of procedures and the progress of labor to the patient and family. Assist with breathing techniques, and offer praise.
- Educate the patient in the latent phase of labor, pain relief measures, and possible ways to distract herself during this portion of labor.

FIRST STAGE OF LABOR—ACTIVE PHASE

- Contractions are moderate to strong, 3 to 5 minutes apart, and more regular; each lasts 40 to 70 seconds.
- Provide fluids and comfort measures such as walking, rocking, water, and frequent position changes. Encourage the patient to void. Assist with breathing techniques, and offer praise and pericare.
- Educate the patient on pain relief measures, including medications.

FIRST STAGE OF LABOR—TRANSITION

- Lasts approximately 20 to 40 minutes; contractions are strong to very strong and 2 to 3 minutes apart; each contraction lasts 45 to 90 seconds.
- Nausea and vomiting, sweating, loss of control, shaking, irritability, hyperventilation, increased bloody show, and the need to push.
- Provide constant support, assist with breathing techniques, provide comfort and pericare, offer medications as needed, and provide fluids.

SECOND STAGE OF LABOR

- Lasts approximately 1 to 3 hours; the urge to push is strong.
- Woman describes a ring of fire as perineum stretches and fetal head crowns.
- Apply warm compresses to perineum to aid with relaxation. Notify the physician and call the nursery if indicated for high-risk fetus.

THIRD STAGE OF LABOR

- Uterus is firm; sudden gush of fluid, lengthening of the umbilical cord, and appearance of the placenta at the vaginal introitus occur.
- Perform fundal massage; administer oxytocic medications as ordered.

FOURTH STAGE OF LABOR

- First 4 hours postpartum begins the last stage of labor.
- Provide fundal massage; assess newborn; woman begins breast-feeding.

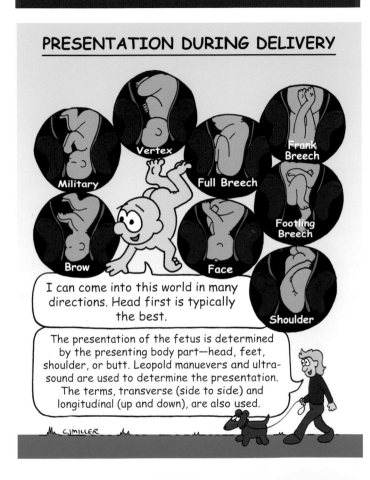

Presentation during Delivery

DEFINITION

- Presentation refers to the part of the fetus that enters the pelvis first with the rest of the fetus following through the birth canal during labor and delivery.
- Presentation can be determined with the use of Leopold maneuvers, which is a series of maneuvers performed on the maternal abdomen and confirmed by abdominal ultrasound.

THREE CATEGORIES OF PRESENTATION

- Cephalic presentation has four variations and is the most common (96% of pregnancies):
  - Vertex: Is the most common type of cephalic presentation; the fetal head is fully flexed; is also called an *occiput presentation*.
  - Military: The head is in a neutral position, neither flexed nor extended.
  - Brow: The fetal head is partly extended. The brow presentation is unstable, usually converting to a vertex presentation if the head flexes or to a face presentation if it extends. The longest supraoccipitomental diameter is presenting.
  - Face: The head is extended, and the fetal occiput is near the fetal spine. The submentobregmatic diameter is presenting.
- Breech: Is more common in preterm births, neonates with hydrocephalus, abnormalities of the maternal uterus and pelvis, and placenta previa.
  - Frank breech: Is the most common variation, occurring when the fetal legs are extended across the abdomen toward the shoulders.
  - Full (complete) breech: Is a reversal of the usual cephalic presentation. The head, knees, and hips are flexed, but the buttocks are presenting.
  - Footling breech: Occurs when one or both feet are presenting.
- Shoulder: Is a transverse lie and may occur with preterm birth, high parity, prematurely ruptured membranes, hydramnios, and placenta previa.

MEDICAL MANAGEMENT

- Vaginal birth (piper forceps, external cephalic version [ECV]), cesarean birth

NURSING IMPLICATIONS

1. Inform the patient about the fetus' presentation.
2. Breech presentation can be complicated with umbilical cord prolapse and head entrapment.
3. Shoulder presentation can also precipitate cord prolapse.
4. Teach the patient with a breech or shoulder presentation about the need for a cesarean delivery.

HYPEREMESIS GRAVIDARUM

- Vomiting
- Dehydration
- Weight loss (>5%)
- Increased pulse rate
- Decreased blood pressure
- Poor skin tugor
- Decreased urine output
- Increased ketones in urine

Patient Education

- Eat small, frequent meals.
- Take recommended over-the-counter and prescription antiemetic medications.
- Report decreased urine output or no voiding in 4 to 6 hours.

I like large, frequent meals.

Hyperemesis Gravidarum

DEFINITION

Hyperemesis gravidarum is persistent, uncontrollable vomiting that begins in the first weeks of pregnancy and may continue throughout the pregnancy.

SIGNS AND SYMPTOMS

- Vomiting, weight loss, dehydration, metabolic acidosis from starvation, and elevated blood and urine ketones
- Alkalosis from the loss of hydrochloric acid in the gastric fluids and hypokalemia

MEDICAL MANAGEMENT

- Antiemetics, such as promethazine (Phenergan), ondansetron (Zofran), metoclopramide (Reglan), methylprednisolone (Medrol), pyridoxine (vitamin B$_6$)
- Intravenous (IV) fluid and electrolyte replacement for severe cases
- Parenteral nutrition for nonresponsive cases to medical treatment

NURSING IMPLICATIONS

1. Dietary: Patient receives nothing by mouth (NPO status) for the first 48 hours; after her condition improves, six small feedings are alternated with liquid nourishment in small amounts every 1 to 2 hours; if vomiting recurs, NPO status is resumed, and administering IV fluids is restarted.
2. Teach woman to sit up after meals to reduce gastric reflux.
3. Monitor for complications associated with fluid loss and acid-base imbalance.

Serious/life-threatening implications	Important nursing implications
Common clinical findings	Patient teaching

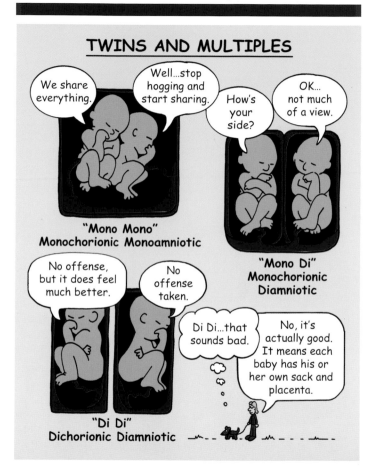

Twins and Multiples

DEFINITION

- Multifetal pregnancies or multiple gestation has been increasing as a result of a rise in maternal age and infertility treatments that induce multiple ovulations.

TYPES

- Monozygotic twins
  - Are conceived by a single sperm and single ovum.
  - Have the same genetic material; a single conceptus divides early in gestation.
  - Are the same gender.
  - May have one or two amnions and one or two chorions.
  - Fertility medications increase the incidence of monozygotic twins.
- Dizygotic twins
  - Are conceived by two ova fertilized by different sperm.
  - May be the same gender or different.
  - May not have similar physical traits.
  - May be hereditary in families.
  - Increases in frequency with maternal age up to 35 years of age, with parity, and with use of fertility medications.
  - Have separate amnions and chorions.
- High multifetal gestation
  - Pregnancy is with triplets or more fetuses.
  - May arise from a single zygote, from a combination of a single and multiple zygotes, or from separate zygotes.
  - Poses greater risks to both mother and fetuses.
  - Incidence of long-term handicaps and disabilities is higher as the number of fetuses increases.

Serious/life-threatening implications	Important nursing implications
Common clinical findings	Patient teaching

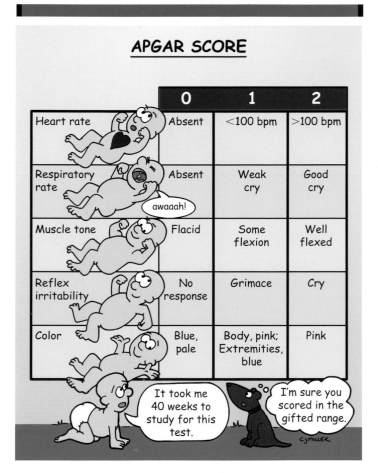

What You Need to Know

APGAR Score

DEFINITION

The APGAR score is the first assessment obtained immediately after birth. Evaluation is made at 1 minute and 5 minutes. It permits a rapid assessment of the newborn's transition to an extrauterine existence based on five signs: (1) heart rate, (2) respiratory rate, (3) muscle tone, (4) reflex irritability, and (5) color. The infant is assigned a score of 0, 1, or 2 in each of the five areas, and the scores are then totaled.

APGAR SCORING

- Heart rate: Is determined by auscultation with a stethoscope or palpation of the umbilical cord.
- Respiratory rate: Is based on the observation of respiratory movement.
- Muscle tone: Is based on the degree of flexion and movement of extremities.
- Reflex irritability: Is based on the response to a bulb aspiration or catheter inserted into the nasopharynx.
- Color: Is determined by generalized skin color described as cyanotic, pallid, or pink.

INTERPRETATION

- Scores of 0 to 3 indicates severe distress.
- Scores of 4 to 6 indicate moderate difficulty.
- Scores of 7 to 10 indicate that the infant is having minimal or no difficulty adjusting to extrauterine life.

NURSING IMPLICATIONS

1. The APGAR score does not predict future physiologic outcomes.
2. It is most useful in describing an infant's transition to the extrauterine environment.
3. If resuscitation is required, it should begin before the 1-minute APGAR evaluation.

| Serious/life-threatening implications | Important nursing implications |
| Common clinical findings | Patient teaching |

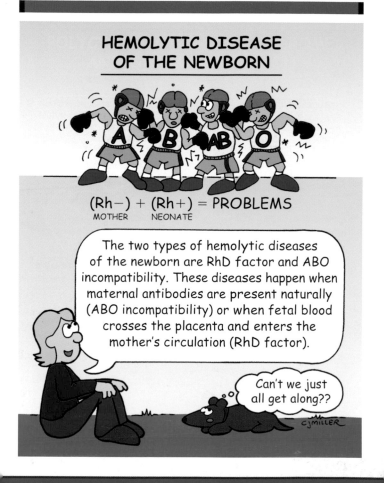

HEMOLYTIC DISEASE OF THE NEWBORN

(Rh−) + (Rh+) = PROBLEMS
MOTHER   NEONATE

The two types of hemolytic diseases of the newborn are RhD factor and ABO incompatibility. These diseases happen when maternal antibodies are present naturally (ABO incompatibility) or when fetal blood crosses the placenta and enters the mother's circulation (RhD factor).

Can't we just all get along??

—— **What You Need to Know** ——

Hemolytic Disease of the Newborn

TYPES

- **ABO incompatibility:** Is more common than Rh incompatibility. It causes less severe problems in the affected infant.
  - ABO incompatibility occurs if the fetal blood type is A, B, or AB and the maternal blood type is O.
  - ABO incompatibility occurs because naturally occurring anti-A and anti-B antibodies are transferred across the placenta to the fetus.
  - First-born infants can be affected.
  - Only occasionally is an exchange transfusion required.
  - Rarely precipitates significant anemia from hemolysis of red blood cells (RBCs).
- **Rh incompatibility:** Is also referred to as isoimmunization.
  - Rh incompatibility occurs when an RhD-negative mother has an RhD-positive fetus who inherits the dominant Rh-positive gene from the father.
  - If the mother is Rh negative and the father is Rh positive and homozygous for the Rh factor, all offspring will be Rh positive. If the father is heterozygous for the Rh factor, a 50% chance exists that each infant born will be Rh positive and a 50% chance exists that each infant will be Rh negative.
  - An Rh-negative fetus is in no danger, because the fetus is the same Rh factor as the mother. Only the Rh-positive infant of an Rh-negative mother is at risk.
  - Erythroblastosis fetalis and hydrops fetalis are complications.

NURSING IMPLICATIONS

1. During the first prenatal visit, the status of an Rh-negative mother is monitored by an indirect Coombs test to determine whether the mother has antibodies to the Rh antigen.
2. An indirect Coombs test is repeated at 28 weeks.
3. Encourage the mother to continue prenatal visits to monitor sensitization status.
4. If no maternal sensitization is found, RhoGAM is given at 28 weeks as a prophylactic measure within 72 hours after the delivery of an Rh-positive infant and after a miscarriage, abortion, or blood transfusion.

Serious/life-threatening implications	Important nursing implications
Common clinical findings	Patient teaching

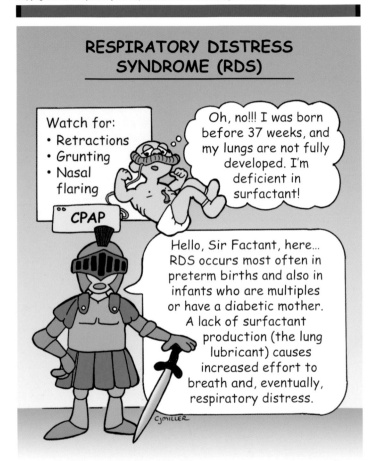

What You Need to Know

Respiratory Distress Syndrome (RDS)

DEFINITION

Respiratory distress syndrome (RDS) is a lung disorder caused by a lack of surfactant, usually affecting preterm infants. A lack of surfactant leads to progressive atelectasis, a loss of functional residual capacity, and a ventilation-perfusion imbalance. By 34 to 36 weeks, the production of surfactant is sufficient to prevent RDS.

RISK FACTORS

- Prematurity

SIGNS AND SYMPTOMS

- Tachypnea, grunting on expiration, nasal flaring, and intercostal or subcostal retractions
- Crackles, decreased breath sounds, pallor, and occasional apnea
- Hypercapnia, respiratory acidosis, hypotension, and shock

MEDICAL MANAGEMENT

- Adequate ventilation and oxygenation via continuous positive airway pressure (CPAP) and oxygen therapy
- Surfactant replacement therapy
- Evaluation of acid-base imbalance

NURSING IMPLICATIONS

1. Observe for early signs of RDS.
2. Maintain a neutral thermal environment.
3. Monitor for common complications—patent ductus arteriosus, broncho-pulmonary dysplasia, and retinopathy of prematurity (ROP) as a result of high levels of oxygen.

| Serious/life-threatening implications | Important nursing implications |
| Common clinical findings | Patient teaching |

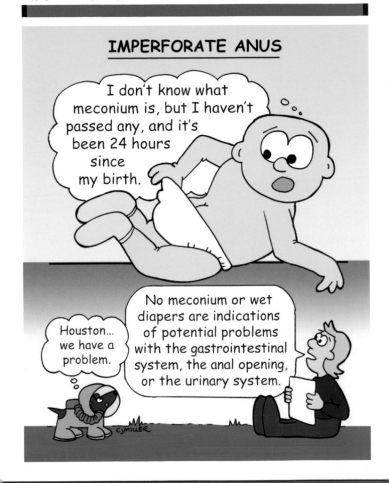

―――――― **What You Need to Know** ――――――

Imperforate Anus

DEFINITION

Imperforate anus is a type of anorectal malformation where the anal opening is not obvious. Many have a fistula from the rectum to the perineum or urinary system.

SIGNS AND SYMPTOMS

- No observable anal opening
- Lack of passage of meconium
- Abdominal distention and vomiting
- If urinary structures are involved (e.g., rectourinary fistula with no anal opening), then meconium may be seen in the urine.

MEDICAL MANAGEMENT

- Treatment is surgical and based on the type of malformation.
- Surgical procedures include anoplasty, colostomy, posterior sagittal anorectoplasty (PSARP), and other pull-through procedures.

NURSING IMPLICATIONS

1. Identification of the anorectal malformation is most important; watch for the first passage of meconium within the first 24 hours after birth.
2. Preoperative care includes nothing by mouth (NPO) status, intravenous (IV) fluids, and gastrointestinal (GI) decompression.
3. Teach parents perineal, wound, and colostomy care as indicated.
4. Toilet training may be delayed after a pull-through procedure. Some children never achieve bowel continence.

Serious/life-threatening implications	Important nursing implications
Common clinical findings	Patient teaching

COMMON BIRTH INJURIES

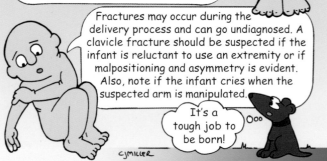

Caput succedaneum is a common scalp lesion. Typically, the swelling extends beyond the bone margins. Don't worry, mom, no treatment is necessary. It will go away in a few days.

Cephalohematoma forms when blood vessels rupture during the delivery process and is most often associated with vacuum-assisted delivery. The involved area does not extend beyond the limits of the bone. No treatment is required, but it may take 2 weeks to 3 months to resolve.

Fractures may occur during the delivery process and can go undiagnosed. A clavicle fracture should be suspected if the infant is reluctant to use an extremity or if malpositioning and asymmetry is evident. Also, note if the infant cries when the suspected arm is manipulated.

It's a tough job to be born!

CJMILLER

─────────── **What You Need to Know** ───────────

Common Birth Injuries

DEFINITION

Many factors can predispose an infant to a birth injury. Many injuries are minor and resolve either spontaneously or with minor intervention. Three common injuries include caput succedaneum, cephalohematoma, and fractured clavicle.

CAPUT SUCCEDANEUM

- Edematous swelling extends beyond the bone margins (sutures) and may have petechiae and ecchymosis.
- **C**rosses **s**utures—think of the letters **c** and **s** in **c**aput **s**uccedaneum.
- Is present at or shortly after birth.
- No specific treatment is necessary.
- Swelling subsides in a few days.
- Teach and reassure parents that the swelling will disappear quickly.

CEPHALOHEMATOMA

- Blood collects between the bone and periosteum when blood vessels rupture during labor or delivery. Blood loss is not significant.
- Is associated with forceps deliveries and vacuum extraction.
- Does not cross the suture lines.
- Swelling is minimally present at birth and increased on the second or third day.
- No treatment is required; absorbs in 2 weeks to 3 months.
- Teach and reassure parents that swelling will subside and that the nature of the swelling is benign.

FRACTURED CLAVICLE

- Is associated with difficult vertex or breech deliveries of large infants.
- May note crepitus and a palpable spongy mass of localized edema and hematoma over clavicle area.
- May also have no symptoms; however, observe for limited used of the affected arm, malposition of the arm, asymmetric reflex, focal swelling or tenderness, or crying when arm is moved.
- Immobilization and the relief of pain are managed by the abduction of the arm on the side of the fractured clavicle at more than 60 degrees with the elbow flexed at more than 90 degrees for 7 to 10 days.

Serious/life-threatening implications	Important nursing implications
Common clinical findings	Patient teaching

INFANTS OF DIABETIC MOTHERS

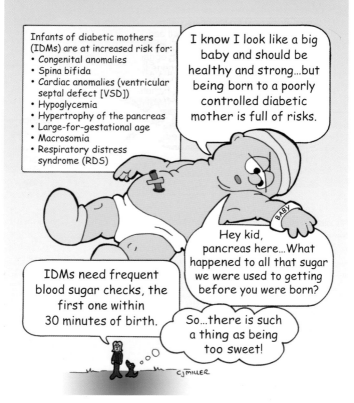

Infants of diabetic mothers (IDMs) are at increased risk for:
- Congenital anomalies
- Spina bifida
- Cardiac anomalies (ventricular septal defect [VSD])
- Hypoglycemia
- Hypertrophy of the pancreas
- Large-for-gestational age
- Macrosomia
- Respiratory distress syndrome (RDS)

I know I look like a big baby and should be healthy and strong...but being born to a poorly controlled diabetic mother is full of risks.

Hey kid, pancreas here...What happened to all that sugar we were used to getting before you were born?

IDMs need frequent blood sugar checks, the first one within 30 minutes of birth.

So...there is such a thing as being too sweet!

—————————— **What You Need to Know** ——————————

Infants of Diabetic Mothers

DEFINITION

The offspring of diabetic mothers are at higher risk for a large number of congenital anomalies. The single most important factor influencing fetal well-being is the mother's normoglycemic status.

RISK FACTORS AFFECTING INFANT SURVIVAL

- Duration of the maternal diabetes before pregnancy
- Age of onset of diabetes
- Extent of vascular complications
- Current problems of pyelonephritis, diabetic ketoacidosis, pregnancy-induced hypertension, and noncompliance

SIGNS AND SYMPTOMS

- Hypoglycemia develops shortly after birth, usually within 1½ to 4 hours, especially in children of mothers with uncontrolled diabetes.
- Physical characteristics include macrosomia, plump, full-faced, and plethoric; has lots of vernix caseosa.
- In mothers with advanced diabetes, the infants may be small for gestational age or have intrauterine growth retardation as a result of placental insufficiency.
- Infant has increased incidence of hypocalcemia, hyperbilirubinemia, hypomagnesemia, and respiratory distress syndrome (RDS).

NURSING IMPLICATIONS

1. Carefully monitor blood sugar after delivery.
2. Monitor for complications of RDS, hyperbilirubinemia, and electrolyte imbalance.
3. Assess infant for anomalies or birth injuries (e.g., fracture clavicle, brachial plexus injury, palsy).
4. Oral intake (breast milk or formula) is started within the first hour after birth if the infant's cardiorespiratory status is stable.
5. Because the infant's hypertrophied pancreas is sensitive to blood glucose levels (as a result of elevated blood sugar levels throughout pregnancy), administering oral glucose may trigger a massive insulin release leading to rebound hypoglycemia.

Serious/life-threatening implications	Important nursing implications
Common clinical findings	Patient teaching

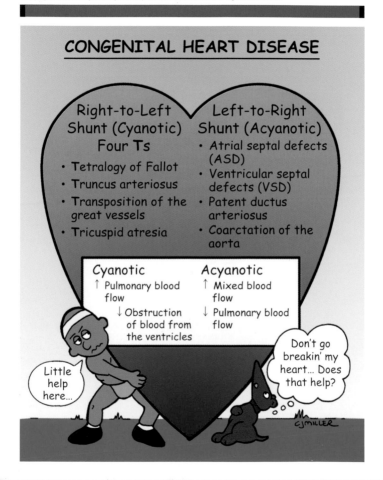

— What You Need to Know —
Congenital Heart Disease

DEFINITION

- Left-to-right shunt (acyanotic): Atrial septal defect, ventricular septal defect (most common anomaly), patent ductus arteriosus, pulmonic stenosis, and coarctation of the aorta
- Right-to-left shunt (cyanotic)—Four Ts: (1) **t**etralogy of Fallot, (2) **t**runcus arteriosus, (3) **t**ransposition of the great arteries, and (4) **t**ricuspid atresia

RISK FACTORS

- Maternal: Diabetes, alcohol consumption, environment toxins, and infections
- Infant: Chromosomal abnormalities, specific syndromes, and other congenital defects

SIGNS AND SYMPTOMS

- Defects with left-to-right shunting cause symptoms of heart failure:
  - Impaired myocardial function: Tachycardia (greater than 160 beats/min), gallop heart rhythm, diaphoresis, easily fatigued, poor exercise tolerance, cold extremities, weak pulses, slow capillary refill, low blood pressure (BP), mottled skin, and extreme pallor or duskiness
  - Pulmonary congestion: Tachypnea (greater than 60 breaths/min in infants), costal retractions, dyspnea on exertion, inability to feed, poor weight gain, orthopnea, wheezing, dry, hacking cough, and gasping and grunting respirations
  - Systemic venous congestion: Hepatomegaly, edema, and weight gain from fluid retention
- Defects that result in decreased pulmonary blood flow cause cyanosis.

MEDICAL MANAGEMENT

- Stabilization with medications—digoxin, angiotensin-converting enzyme (ACE) inhibitors, diuretics, and beta blockers
- Surgical repair of the defect

NURSING IMPLICATIONS

1. Nursing interventions for infants are different from those for older children.
2. Monitor for the development of heart failure.
3. Decrease cardiac demands—promote rest, and plan feeding to accommodate the infant's sleep and wake pattern.
4. Reduce respiratory distress—elevate head and administer oxygen.
5. Maintain nutritional status.
6. Teach family about medications and the signs of heart failure.

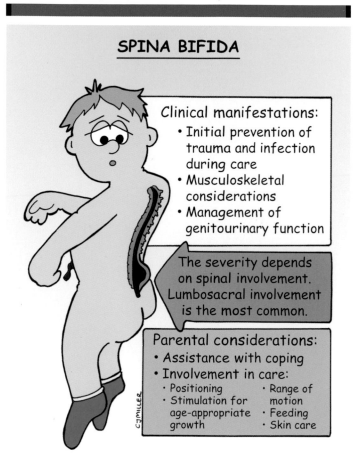

SPINA BIFIDA

Clinical manifestations:
- Initial prevention of trauma and infection during care
- Musculoskeletal considerations
- Management of genitourinary function

The severity depends on spinal involvement. Lumbosacral involvement is the most common.

Parental considerations:
- Assistance with coping
- Involvement in care:
  - Positioning
  - Stimulation for age-appropriate growth
  - Range of motion
  - Feeding
  - Skin care

CJMILLER

— **What You Need to Know** —

Spina Bifida

DEFINITION

The most common defect of the central nervous system is **spina bifida**, which is a defect in the closure of the osseous (bony) spine. *Spina bifida occulta* and *spina bifida cystica* are the two types of spina bifida.

RISK FACTORS

- Multifactorial: Drugs, radiation, maternal malnutrition, chemicals, and possible genetic mutation in folate pathways.

SIGNS AND SYMPTOMS

- Spina bifida occulta: Defect is not visible externally; it is located in lumbo-sacral area (L5 and S1). It may not be apparent unless cutaneous manifestations (e.g., skin depression or dimple, nevi, tuft of hair) or neuromuscular manifestations (e.g., progressive disturbance of gait with foot weakness, bowel and bladder sphincter disturbances) are evident.
- Spina bifida cystica: Defect is visible with an external saclike protrusion. It has two major forms—*meningocele* (meninges and spinal fluid are encased) and *myelomeningocele* (meninges, spinal fluid, and nerves are encased).
  - Below the second lumbar vertebra: Flaccid, partial paralysis of lower extremities, sensory deficit, overflow incontinence with constant dribbling of urine, lack of bowel control, and sometimes rectal prolapse
  - Below the third sacral vertebrae: No motor impairment exists. Saddle anesthesia with bladder and anal sphincter paralysis may be present.

MEDICAL MANAGEMENT

- Early surgical closure of myelomeningocele sac

NURSING IMPLICATIONS

1. Assess the intactness of the sac at birth, and prevent trauma.
2. Assess the level of neurologic involvement.
3. Monitor urinary output and passage of meconium.
4. Place the infant in an incubator. Apply sterile, moist, and nonadherent dressings over defect; usually use normal saline solution.
5. Avoid measuring the rectal temperature; a thermometer can cause irritation of existing bowel sphincter dysfunction.
6. Place the infant in a prone or partial side-lying position after surgery.
7. Teach parents regarding positioning, feeding, skin and wound care, and range-of-motion (ROM) exercises.

HYDROCEPHALUS

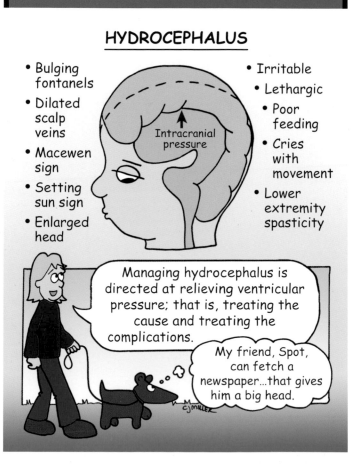

━━━━━━━━━━━ What You Need to Know ━━━━━━━━━━━

Hydrocephalus

DEFINITION

Hydrocephalus is a condition caused by an imbalance in the production and absorption of cerebrospinal fluid (CSF) in the ventricular system.

TYPES

- Nonobstructive or communicating: The absorption of the CSF in the subarachnoid space is impaired.
- Obstructive or noncommunicating: The flow of the CSF through the ventricular system is obstructed.

  Note: The terms *communicating* and *noncommunicating* traditionally refer to nonobstructive and obstructive types when pneumoencephalography is used to establish a diagnosis. Because other diagnostic methods are now used, these terms may be only reference points in the diagnosis.

SIGNS AND SYMPTOMS

- Infancy (early)
  - Abnormally rapid head growth; bulging, tense, and nonpulsatile fontanels
  - Separated sutures and dilated scalp veins
  - Macewen sign (cracked-pot sound on percussion) due to thinning bones
- Infancy (late)
  - Frontal protrusion or enlargement (frontal bossing) and depressed eyes
  - Setting sun sign (sclera visible above the iris) and sluggish pupils with unequal response to light
- Infancy (general)
  - Irritability, lethargy, and change in the level of consciousness (LOC)
  - Opisthotonos (often extreme); lower extremity spasticity; shrill, brief, high-pitched cry
- Childhood
  - Headache on awakening and improvement after vomiting or maintaining an upright posture; papilledema, strabismus, ataxia, irritability, and lethargy

NURSING IMPLICATIONS

1. Record daily occipitofrontal circumference measurements (OFC) at the point of the largest measurement. Mark areas on the head with a pen to ensure consistent placement of the tape for measuring.
2. Postoperative shunt insertion: Position the patient on the unoperative side to prevent pressure on the shunt valve; position is flat; watch for neurologic signs and abdominal distention.
3. Teach the family the signs of shunt malfunction; advise no contact sports, and recommend a helmet for play.

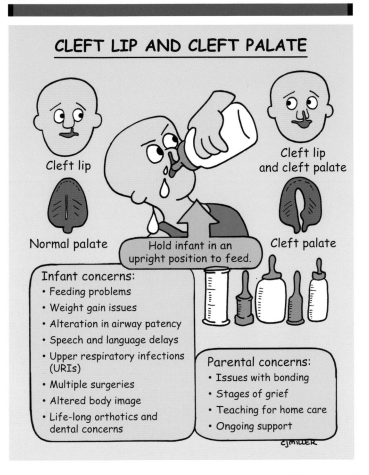

CLEFT LIP AND CLEFT PALATE

Cleft lip

Cleft lip and cleft palate

Normal palate

Cleft palate

Hold infant in an upright position to feed.

Infant concerns:
- Feeding problems
- Weight gain issues
- Alteration in airway patency
- Speech and language delays
- Upper respiratory infections (URIs)
- Multiple surgeries
- Altered body image
- Life-long orthotics and dental concerns

Parental concerns:
- Issues with bonding
- Stages of grief
- Teaching for home care
- Ongoing support

cjmiller

━━━ What You Need to Know ━━━
Cleft Lip and Cleft Palate

DEFINITION

Cleft lip (CL) is a fissure of the upper lip, which may vary from a slight notch to a complete separation or cleft extending into the nostril; it may be unilateral or bilateral. A cleft lip is caused by a failure of the maxillary and median nasal processes to fuse early in fetal life.

Cleft palate (CP) is a midline fissure of the palate that results from a failure of the two sides to fuse; it may involve the soft and hard palates.

SIGNS AND SYMPTOMS

- CL: Is visible at birth; dental anomalies are evident; feeding and weight gain problems exist before repair.
- CP: Feeding difficulties (risk of aspiration) are present; growth failure and speech problems exist.

MEDICAL MANAGEMENT

- Surgical repair—CL at 3 months; CP at 9 to 15 months

NURSING IMPLICATIONS

1. Assess for CL (visible) and CP (palpate the palate with gloved finger during newborn assessment).
2. Postoperative care for CL: Protect the suture line; position the patient on the right side or upright in an infant seat (avoid the prone position); avoid the use of suction or objects in the mouth such as a tongue depressor, thermometer, spoon, or straws to avoid trauma to the healing suture line.
3. CL special feeding: Use a slow-flow nipple, plastic squeezable bottle, and Haberman feeder until the suture line heals.
4. Postoperative care for CP: Use a feeding cup, syringe feeding, Haberman feeder, or Breck feeder; avoid spoon and fork. The child may lie on the abdomen, especially immediately after surgery.
5. Teach parents to get their infant accustomed to a care and feeding method (possibly use of a cup) during the postoperative period.

Serious/life-threatening implications	Important nursing implications
Common clinical findings	Patient teaching

HYPERBILIRUBINEMIA

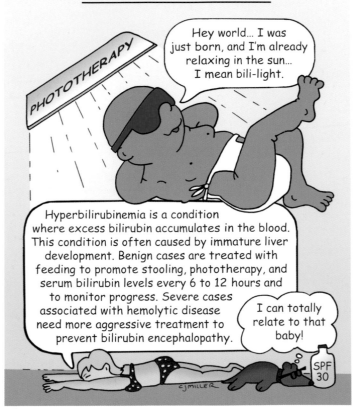

--- **What You Need to Know** ---

Hyperbilirubinemia

DEFINITION

Hyperbilirubinemia refers to an excessive level of unconjugated bilirubin in the blood and is characterized by jaundice. It is a common finding in newborns that is usually benign.

ETIOLOGY

- Physiologic jaundice: Immature hepatic function plus increased bilirubin load from red blood cell (RBC) hemolysis
- Breast-feeding–associated jaundice (early onset): Decreased milk intake related to fewer calories consumed by the infant before the mother's milk is well established
- Breast milk jaundice (late onset): Possible factors in breast milk that prevent bilirubin conjugation; less frequent stooling
- Hemolytic disease: Blood antigen incompatibility causing hemolysis of large numbers of RBCs

SIGNS AND SYMPTOMS

- Physiologic jaundice: Onset is after 24 hours; it peaks in 3 to 4 days and declines in 5 to 7 days.
- Breast-feeding–associated jaundice (early onset): Onset is in 2 to 4 days; it peaks in 3 to 5 days with variable duration.
- Breast milk jaundice (late onset): Onset is on the fourth day; it peaks in 10 to 15 days and jaundice may remain for 3 to 12 weeks.
- Hemolytic disease: Onset is within the first 24 hours (levels increase by >5 mg/dl/day).

LABORATORY FINDINGS

- Newborn: Levels must exceed 5 mg/dl before jaundice is observable. (Normal value of unconjugated bilirubin is 0.2 to 1.4 mg/dl.)

MEDICAL MANAGEMENT

- Phototherapy (lights, fiberoptic blankets)

NURSING IMPLICATIONS

1. Cover the eyes and genitalia while under the light. Frequently reposition the patient to expose all body surface areas to the light.
2. Accurately chart the time spent under light. Check the eyes every 4 to 6 hours for evidence of discharge, excessive pressure, or corneal ulceration.
3. Teach the parents about home phototherapy if ordered.

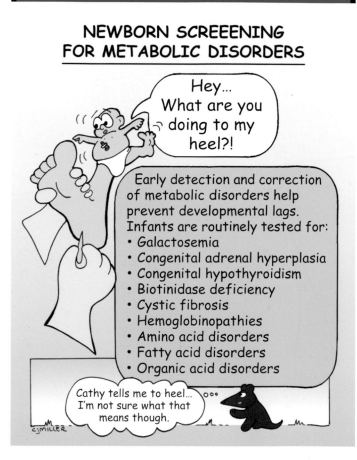

━━━━━━━━━━━━━━ **What You Need to Know** ━━━━━━━━━━━━━━

Newborn Screening for Metabolic Disorders

DEFINITION

Newborn screening tests are performed to assess for serious developmental, genetic, and metabolic disorders so that early diagnosis and treatment can be initiated during the critical time before symptoms develop. Most of these illnesses are very rare.

Individual states regulate newborn screening, so the diseases for which newborns are screened vary considerably from state to state. The most thorough screening panel checks for about 40 disorders. All 50 states screen for congenital hypothyroidism, galactosemia, and phenylketonuria (PKU).

LABORATORY FINDINGS

• Normal values for each screening test may vary depending on how the test is performed.

NURSING IMPLICATIONS

1. Heel stick is the primary method to obtain a blood sample.
2. Warm the heel with an application of warm water 10 to 15 minutes before the procedure.
3. Use an automatic puncture device; it causes less pain. Avoid using manual lance blades in newborns.
4. Use the outer aspect of the heel and an automatic device that goes no deeper than 2.4 mm.
5. To identify the appropriate puncture site, draw an imaginary line running from between the fourth and fifth toes and parallel to the lateral aspect of the foot to the heel where the stick should be made. A second line can also be drawn from the great toe to the medial aspect of the heel to identify another lateral site on the heel to puncture.
6. Fill all circles on the metabolic screening form with blood.
7. Necrotizing osteochondritis from a lancet penetration of the bone is a serious complication after a heel stick.
8. Teach parents the importance of having a newborn screening test and a follow-up appointment for the results.

| Serious/life-threatening implications | Important nursing implications |
| Common clinical findings | Patient teaching |

NEONATAL ABSTINENCE SYNDROME

Signs of withdrawal:

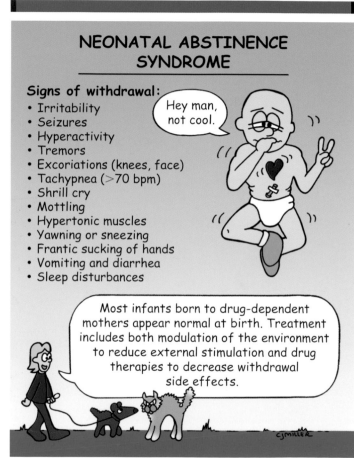

- Irritability
- Seizures
- Hyperactivity
- Tremors
- Excoriations (knees, face)
- Tachypnea (>70 bpm)
- Shrill cry
- Mottling
- Hypertonic muscles
- Yawning or sneezing
- Frantic sucking of hands
- Vomiting and diarrhea
- Sleep disturbances

Most infants born to drug-dependent mothers appear normal at birth. Treatment includes both modulation of the environment to reduce external stimulation and drug therapies to decrease withdrawal side effects.

--- **What You Need to Know** ---

Neonatal Abstinence Syndrome

DEFINITION

Neonatal abstinence syndrome (NAS) is a group of problems that occur in a newborn who was exposed to addictive illegal or prescription drugs while in utero, such as amphetamines, barbiturates, cocaine, diazepam, marijuana, opiates (e.g., heroin, methadone, codeine), and alcohol. The drugs pass through the placenta, and the infant becomes addicted along with the mother. At birth, the infant is still dependent on the drug. Because the infant is no longer getting the drug after birth, symptoms of withdrawal occur.

SIGNS AND SYMPTOMS

- Increased muscle tone and respiratory rate
- Disturbed sleep; fever; excessive sucking; and loose watery, stools
- Projectile vomiting, mottling, crying, nasal stuffiness, and hyperactive Moro reflex
- Sucks avidly on fists; displays exaggerated rooting reflex, but tends to be a poor feeder
- Generalized perspiring

NURSING IMPLICATIONS

1. Reduce external stimuli (e.g., dim lights, reduce noise levels) that might trigger hyperactivity and irritability; place the infant in side-lying position with legs flexed.
2. Provide adequate nutrition and hydration; providing care on demand rather than on a fixed schedule works best for these infants.
3. Teach the mother to wrap her infant snuggly and rock; holding the infant helps ease withdrawal and distress.
4. Degree of withdrawal is closely related to the amount of the drug the mother has habitually taken, the length of time she has been taking the drug, and her drug level at delivery.
5. The nearer to delivery that the mother takes the drug, the longer it takes the infant to show signs of withdrawal.
6. Protect the extremities, elbows, and cheeks from skin abrasions caused by the hyperactive infant rubbing on bed linens.

| Serious/life-threatening implications | Important nursing implications |
| Common clinical findings | Patient teaching |

GYNECOLOGIC TERMS

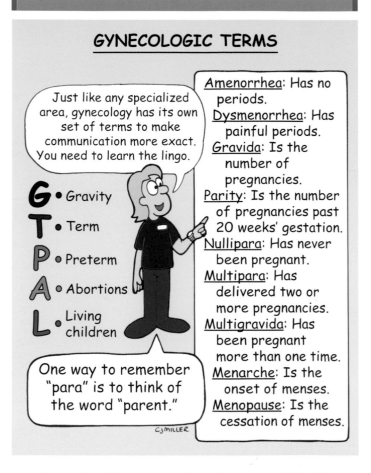

Just like any specialized area, gynecology has its own set of terms to make communication more exact. You need to learn the lingo.

G • Gravity
T • Term
P • Preterm
A • Abortions
L • Living children

One way to remember "para" is to think of the word "parent."

Amenorrhea: Has no periods.
Dysmenorrhea: Has painful periods.
Gravida: Is the number of pregnancies.
Parity: Is the number of pregnancies past 20 weeks' gestation.
Nullipara: Has never been pregnant.
Multipara: Has delivered two or more pregnancies.
Multigravida: Has been pregnant more than one time.
Menarche: Is the onset of menses.
Menopause: Is the cessation of menses.

What You Need to Know

Gynecologic Terms

DEFINITION OF TERMS

Being familiar with common gynecologic terms used to describe pregnancy, the pregnant woman, and gynecologic issues is important.

- **Amenorrhea:** Absence or suppression of menses
- **Dysmenorrhea:** Painful menstrual periods
- **Gravida:** Woman who is pregnant or has been pregnant; is the number of pregnancies
- **Menarche:** Onset of beginning of menstrual periods
- **Menopause:** Permanent cessation of menstrual cycle; diagnosed after 1 year without menses
- **Multigravida:** Woman who has had two or more pregnancies; is the number of pregnancies
- **Multipara:** Woman who has completed two or more pregnancies to 20 or more weeks' gestation
- **Nullipara:** Woman who has never been pregnant
- **Parity:** Number of pregnancies in which the fetus or fetuses have reached 20 weeks' gestation when born, not the number of fetuses (e.g., twins) born; whether the fetus is born alive or is stillborn (i.e., fetus who shows no signs of life at birth) does not affect parity
- **Postdate** or **postterm:** Pregnancy that goes beyond 42 weeks' gestation
- **Preterm:** Pregnancy that has reached 20 weeks' gestation but ends before the completion of 37 weeks' gestation
- **Primigravida:** Woman who is pregnant for the first time
- **Primipara:** Woman who has completed one pregnancy with a fetus or fetuses who have reached 20 weeks' gestation
- **Viability:** Capacity to live outside the uterus; approximately 22 to 25 weeks' gestation

GTPAL SYSTEM

The acronym **GTPAL** (**g**ravidity, **t**erm, **p**reterm, **a**bortions, **l**iving children) may be helpful in noting pregnancy outcomes. For example, for the woman who has been pregnant twice, had her first pregnancy end with a miscarriage at 20 weeks, gives birth at week 33, and the neonate survives, the GTPAL abbreviation that represents this information is 2-0-1-1-1. During her next pregnancy, the abbreviation is 3-0-1-1-1 until the infant is born.

Serious/life-threatening implications	Important nursing implications
Common clinical findings	Patient teaching

MENSTRUAL CALENDAR

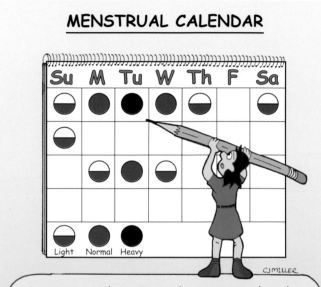

A woman can have irregular menstrual cycles at any time during her reproductive years. Keeping a record of spotting, as well as normal and heavy flow days, can assist the health care provider to make a diagnosis and plan of care. Heavy bleeding can lead to anemia and can be a symptom of uterine fibroids or cancer.

—————— **What You Need to Know** ——————

Menstrual Calendar

DEFINITION

The *menstrual calendar* is a method for women to record spotting, normal flow days, and heavy flow days in an effort to provide a comprehensive picture of monthly bleeding to assist the health care provider in making a plan of care. Irregularities or problems with the menstrual period are among the most common concerns of women and often cause them to seek help from the health care system.

COMMON MENSTRUAL DISORDERS

- Amenorrhea
- Dysmenorrhea
- Premenstrual syndrome
- Endometriosis
- Menorrhagia
- Metrorrhagia

SIGNS AND SYMPTOMS

- Normal menstrual patterns are averages, based on observations and reports from large groups of healthy women.
- Menstrual frequency stabilizes at 28 days within 1 to 2 years after puberty, with a range from 26 to 34 days.
  - No woman's cycle is exactly the same length every month.
  - Typical month-to-month variation in a woman's cycle is usually plus or minus 2 days.
- Menstrual cycle length is most irregular at the extremes of the reproductive years, when anovulatory cycles are most common.
  - Two years after menarche
  - Five years before menopause
- Irregular bleeding, both in length of cycle and amount, occurs often in early adolescence.
  - An average of 20 cycles before ovulation occurs regularly.
  - Cycle lengths of 15 to 45 days are not unusual.
  - Intervals of 3 to 6 months between menses can be normal.
- Typical length of menstrual cycle is approximately 40 years.

NURSING IMPLICATIONS

1. Teach the woman how to use the calendar coding system to track bleeding.
2. Provide simple explanations and counseling about concerns regarding bleeding patterns.

Serious/life-threatening implications	Important nursing implications
Common clinical findings	Patient teaching

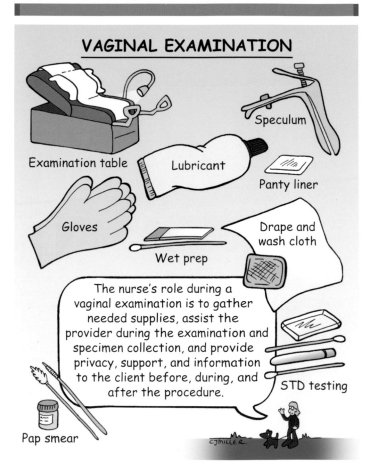

VAGINAL EXAMINATION

Examination table

Speculum

Lubricant

Panty liner

Gloves

Drape and wash cloth

Wet prep

The nurse's role during a vaginal examination is to gather needed supplies, assist the provider during the examination and specimen collection, and provide privacy, support, and information to the client before, during, and after the procedure.

STD testing

Pap smear

━━━━━━━━━━━━━ **What You Need to Know** ━━━━━━━━━━━━━

Vaginal Examination

PROCEDURE

- Explain the procedure to the woman. Ask her to undress, remove her underwear, and put on the gown.
- Ask the woman to empty her bladder before the examination. If needed, explain how to collect a clean-catch urine specimen.
- Wash hands and assemble equipment.
- Position the woman in lithotomy position.
  - Hips and knees are flexed, the buttocks are at the edge of the table, and the heel or knee stirrups support the feet.
  - The woman may prefer to keep her shoes or socks on, especially if the stirrups are not padded.
- Warm the speculum in warm water if a prewarmed one is not available.
- Ask the patient to bear down when the speculum is being inserted.
- Apply gloves and assist the health care provider with the collection of laboratory specimens.
- Have the tube of lubricant open, and apply to the health care provider's fingers with water or a water-soluble lubricant before the bimanual examination.
- When the examination is over, assist the patient to a sitting position and then to a standing position.
- Provide tissues to wipe the lubricant from the perineum.
- Provide privacy for the woman while she is dressing.

NURSING IMPLICATIONS

1. Encourage the patient to use relaxation techniques.
2. Encourage the woman to become involved with the examination if she shows an interest (e.g., by offering a mirror so she can see the area being examined).
3. Monitor for and treat the signs of supine hypotension.
4. Women prefer not to respond to questions until they are upright and at eye level with the examiner.
5. Teach the patient about the importance of regular vulvar self-examination (VSE).

Serious/life-threatening implications	Important nursing implications
Common clinical findings	Patient teaching

"THREE Ls" OF CULTURAL CONSIDERATIONS

Look—Look at your client. Watch her body language, and maintain eye contact.

Listen—Listen to your client, not only to the words that are said but those that are unsaid. Answer questions. Allow the client to feel she is in control of the experience.

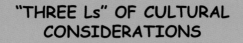

CJMILLER

Learn—Learn from what you have seen and heard. Apply this knowledge to your nursing professionalism. Adapt measures to meet needs, regardless of age, race, religion, or culture.

──── What You Need to Know ────

"Three Ls" of Cultural Considerations

Nurses need to be aware of cultural considerations when working with women and childbearing families. Using the three Ls—look, listen, and learn—can help the nurse provide culturally competent care.

CULTURAL COMPETENCE

The culturally competent nurse has an enhanced ability to provide quality care, which fosters better patient understanding of the plan of care.

CULTURE—A NURSING APPROACH

Consider your own cultural biases and how they affect your nursing care.
Understand the need to recognize cultural implications in planning and implementing nursing care.
Learn how to use cultural assessment tools.
Treat patients with dignity and respect.
Use sensitivity in providing culturally competent care.
Recognize the opportunities to provide specific culture-based nursing care.
Evaluate your own previous encounters with patients from other cultures and backgrounds.

(Reprinted with permission. Zerwekh J, Claborn J: *CULTURE: A mnemonic for assessing and improving cultural competence,* Ingram, Tex, 2006, Nursing Education Consultants.)

QUESTIONS

The following questions elicit cultural expectations about childbearing:
1. What do you and your family think you should do to remain healthy during pregnancy?
2. What can you do or not do to improve your health and the health of your baby?
3. Who do you want with you during labor?
4. What can he or she do to help you be most comfortable during labor?
5. What actions are important for you and your family after the baby's birth?
6. What do you and your family expect from the nurses caring for you?
7. How will family members participate in your pregnancy, childbirth, and parenting?

(From Lowdermilk DL, Perry SE: *Maternity & women's health care,* ed 10, St Louis, 2012, Elsevier–Mosby.)

Serious/life-threatening implications | Important nursing implications
Common clinical findings | Patient teaching

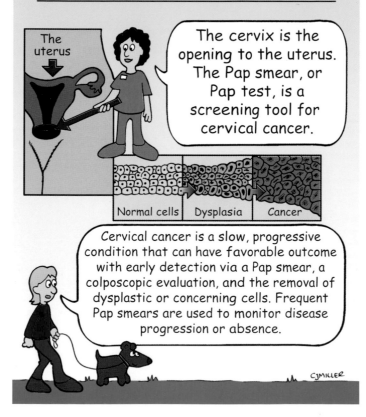

SCREENING FOR CERVICAL CANCER

The uterus

The cervix is the opening to the uterus. The Pap smear, or Pap test, is a screening tool for cervical cancer.

Normal cells | Dysplasia | Cancer

Cervical cancer is a slow, progressive condition that can have favorable outcome with early detection via a Pap smear, a colposcopic evaluation, and the removal of dysplastic or concerning cells. Frequent Pap smears are used to monitor disease progression or absence.

CJMILLER

━━━━━━━━━━━━━━ **What You Need to Know** ━━━━━━━━━━━━━━

Screening for Cervical Cancer

The Bethesda System describes Pap test results.

- Normal (negative) result: No signs of cancer or precancerous cell are found.
- Squamous intraepithelial lesion (SIL): Describes precancerous changes seen in the cells of the cervix. SIL can be low grade (LSIL) or high grade (HSIL). These grades are related to the grades of dysplasia and cervical intraepithelial neoplasia (CIN) (see box). Carcinoma in situ (CIS) is a severe form of HSIL and most likely will progress to cancer.
- Atypical squamous cells; cannot exclude HSIL (ASC-H): Changes in the cervical cells have been found. These changes are not clearly HSIL, but they could be. Further testing is needed.
- Atypical squamous cells of undetermined significance (ASC-US): Is the most common abnormal finding of a Pap test.
- Atypical glandular cells (AGC): Cell changes are found that suggest a precancerous condition of the upper part of the cervix or uterus.

CIN or dysplasia: Describes the actual changes in the cervical cells.

Term	CIN	SIL
Mild dysplasia	1	Low grade
Moderate dysplasia	2	High grade
Severe dysplasia	3	High grade
CIN	3	High grade

Source: American College of Obstetricians and Gynecologists: *Understanding abnormal Pap results,* Washington DC, 2009, The College. Retrieved from http://www.acog.org/publications/patient_education/bp161.cfm

NURSING IMPLICATIONS

1. Pap test specimen is obtained during a pelvic examination. Assemble required materials and explain the procedure to the patient.
2. Guidelines from the American College of Obstetricians and Gynecologists recommend that women begin Pap test screening at age 21 years, be screened every 2 years through age 30 years, and then be screened every 3 years as long as their last three test results have been normal.
3. Teach women who have been vaccinated against HPVs that they still need to have Pap tests.
4. For women 21 years and older with ASC-US, the test is given every 6 months until two normal results occur. The woman can then return to the routine schedule for Pap test screening. For women 20 years and younger with ASC-US or LSIL, the Pap test is repeated annually.

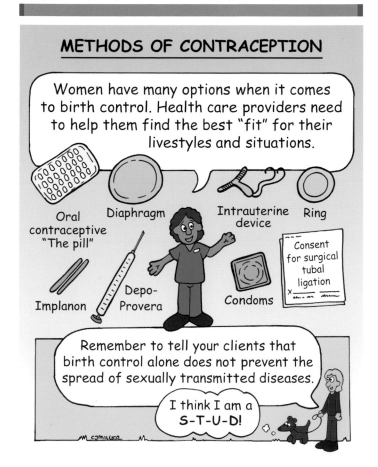

What You Need to Know

Methods of Contraception

- Coitus interruptus: The man withdraws his entire penis from the woman's vagina and moves away from her external genitalia before he ejaculates.
- Failure rate is approximately 27%.

FERTILITY AWARENESS METHODS (FAMs)

- FAMs depend on identifying the beginning and end of the fertile period.
- FAMs include natural family planning; the calendar rhythm, standard days, TwoDay, ovulation, and symptothermal methods; and the home predictor test kits for ovulation. Typical failure rate for most FAMs is 25%.

BARRIER METHODS

- Spermicide: Uses nonoxynol-9 (N-9) to reduce sperm motility. Typical failure rate is 29%.
- Male condom: Thin sheath of rubber is fitted over an erect penis. Typical failure rate is 15%.
- Female condom: Lubricated polyurethane sheath with flexible rings at both ends is inserted in the vagina. Typical failure rate is 21%.

DIAPHRAGMS, CERVICAL CAPS, AND SPONGES

- Diaphragm: Dome-shaped rubber device is fitted over the cervix.
- Cervical cap: Silicone cup or cap is placed over the cervix.
- Contraceptive sponge: Polyurethane sponge containing N-9 spermicide is fitted over the cervix.

HORMONAL METHODS

- Oral contraceptives—Estrogen-progestin or progestin-only pills. Almost all failures are caused by the omission of one or more pills.
- Transdermal contraceptive: A patch is applied to the body.
- Vaginal contraceptive ring: Is inserted into the vagina and delivers continuous hormones.
- Injectable progestin: Is administered intramuscularly (IM) every 3 months.
- Implantable progestin: Is effective for up to 3 years.

INTRAUTERINE DEVICES (IUD)

- Copper device is inserted into the uterus and is effective for 10 years.
- Hormonal system is inserted into the uterus and is effective for 5 years.

EMERGENCY CONTRACEPTION

- Is available without a prescription to any woman over 18 years of age.
- Should be taken no longer than 120 hours after unprotected intercourse or birth control mishap.

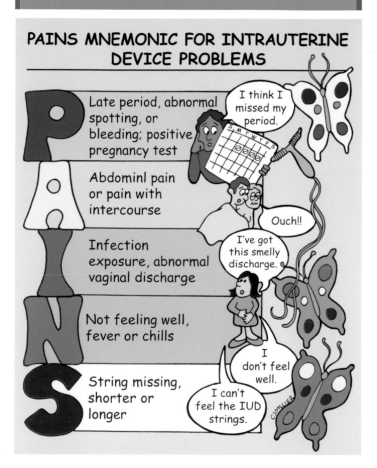

--- **What You Need to Know** ---

PAINS Mnemonic for Intrauterine Device Problems

DEFINITION

An intrauterine device (IUD) is a small T-shaped device used for contraception with bendable arms for insertion through the cervix. It adversely affects sperm motility and irritates the uterus lining, preventing fertilization. Two types are the ParaGard Copper T 380A and the hormonal intrauterine system (Mirena).

ADVANTAGES

- Long-term protection from pregnancy is provided with an immediate return to fertility when the IUD is removed.
- Women who are in mutually monogamous relationships are the best candidates for using an IUD.

DISADVANTAGES

- Increases the risk for pelvic inflammatory disease (PID) after placement.
- Unintentional expulsion of the device, infection, and possible uterine perforation may occur.
- Offers no protection against human immunodeficiency virus (HIV) or other sexually transmitted infections (STIs).

MNEMONIC FOR POTENTIAL COMPLICATIONS

Signs of potential complications related to IUDs can be remembered by:
- **P**eriod late, abnormal spotting or bleeding
- **A**bdominal pain, pain with intercourse
- **I**nfection exposure, abnormal vaginal discharge
- **N**ot feeling well, fever, or chills
- **S**tring missing, shorter or longer

(From Zieman M, Hatcher R, Cwiak C, et al: *A pocket guide to managing contraception,* Tiger, Ga, 2007, Bridging the Gap Foundation.)

NURSING IMPLICATIONS

1. Teach the woman to check for the presence of the IUD string after menstruation to rule out expulsion of the device.
2. Teach the woman that if pregnancy occurs with the IUD in place, she should contact her health care provider and anticipate an ultrasound to confirm that an ectopic pregnancy has not occurred.
3. If pregnant, early removal of the IUD helps decrease the risk of spontaneous miscarriage or preterm labor.
4. In some women who are allergic to copper, a rash develops, necessitating the removal of the copper-bearing IUD.
5. Teach the signs of potential complications using the PAINS mnemonic.

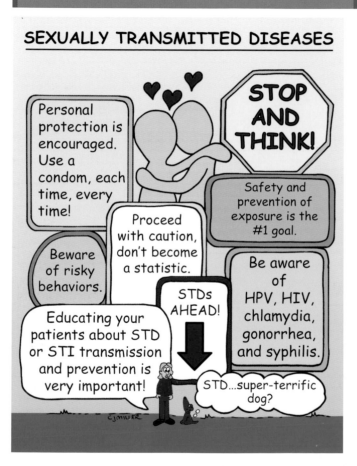

─── **What You Need to Know** ───

Sexually Transmitted Diseases

DEFINITION

Sexually transmitted diseases (STDs) or *sexually transmitted infections* (STIs) are infectious diseases transmitted most commonly through sexual contact, but they can be congenitally acquired. STDs during pregnancy are responsible for significant morbidity and mortality; they can lead to infertility and sterility and can affect a neonate's length and quality of life.

TYPES OF STDs AND CAUSATIVE ORGANISMS

- Chlamydial infection—*Chlamydia trachomatis*
- Gonorrhea—*Neisseria gonorrhoeae*
- Syphilis—*Treponema pallidum*
- Genital herpes—herpes simplex virus (HSV); usually type 2 (HSV-2)
- Genital warts (*Condylomata acuminate*)—human papillomavirus (HPV)

NURSING IMPLICATIONS

1. Teach the patient to take all antibiotic medications, even if symptoms subside in a couple of days.
2. Instruct the patient about hygienic measures, such as washing and urinating after intercourse to flush out some organisms.
3. Teach the importance of the need to treat sexual partners.
4. Many STDs are reportable to the state health department.
5. Encourage sexual abstinence during the communicable phase of the disease.
6. Explain the importance of follow-up examination and reculture to confirm a complete cure.
7. Teach the patient about the symptoms of complications and medication side effects.
8. Teach the patient about precautions to take to avoid contracting an STD:
   - Monogamous partners
   - Avoidance of intercourse with partners who use intravenous (IV) drugs or who have visible lesions in the perineal and oral areas
   - Use of condoms
   - Voiding and washing genitals after coitus to reduce the occurrence of reinfection

---

Serious/life-threatening implications	Important nursing implications
Common clinical findings	Patient teaching

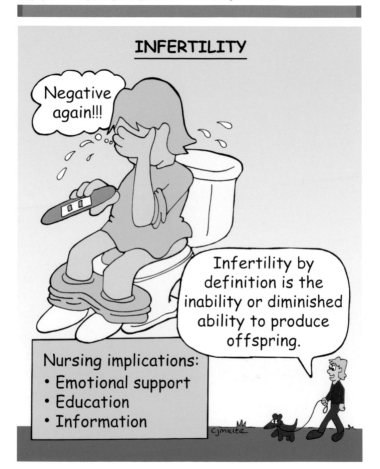

What You Need to Know

Infertility

DEFINITION

Infertility refers to a prolonged time to conceive; sterility means an inability to conceive.

RISK FACTORS

- Female factors: Anovulation; uterine, tubal, or peritoneal problems (endometriosis, chronic pelvic infections); obesity; thyroid dysfunction
- Male factors: Structural or hormonal disorders (undescended testes, hypospadias, varicocele, low testosterone levels, retrograde ejaculation); obesity; medications

MEDICAL MANAGEMENT

- Medical
  - Diagnostic testing: Hormone analysis, ultrasonography, hysterosalpingography, endometrial biopsy, and semen analysis
  - Infertility medications: Clomiphene (Clomid), human menopausal gonadotropin (hMG), follicle-stimulating hormone (FSH), human chorionic gonadotropin (hCG), and gonadotropin-releasing hormone (GnRH)
- Surgical: Reconstructive surgery, chemocautery or thermocautery, cryosurgery, laparoscopy, conization of the cervix, and repair of varicocele
- Reproductive alternatives: In vitro fertilization embryo transfer (IVF-ET), gamete intrafallopian transfer (GIFT), zygote intrafallopian transfer (ZIFT), oocyte donation, embryo donation, therapeutic donor insemination (TDI), surrogate motherhood, and adoption

NURSING IMPLICATIONS

1. Assess the couple's current level of understanding of the factors that promote conception.
2. Provide information regarding the factors that promote conception.
3. Explain basic infertility testing and infertility medication management.
4. Provide support and promote coping, related to the difficulties encountered related to infertility.

| Serious/life-threatening implications | Important nursing implications |
| Common clinical findings | Patient teaching |

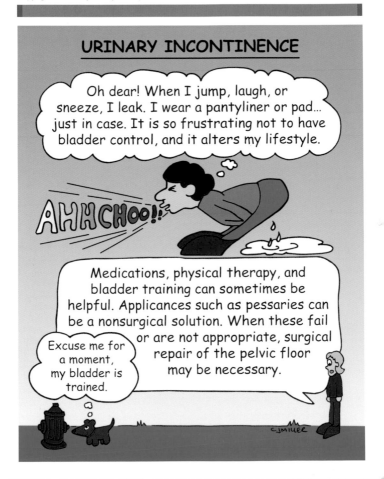

What You Need to Know

Urinary Incontinence

DEFINITION

Urinary incontinence is the loss of bladder control and is a common and often embarrassing problem.

RISK FACTORS

- Overweight, history of hysterectomy, aging
- Multiparity, renal disease, diabetes

SIGNS AND SYMPTOMS

- **Stress incontinence:** Is the loss of urine as a result of an increase in intra-abdominal pressure on the bladder when coughing, sneezing, laughing, exercising, or lifting something heavy. It occurs when the sphincter muscle of the bladder is weakened.
- **Urge incontinence:** Is a sudden, intense urge to urinate, followed by an involuntary loss of urine. The bladder muscle contracts and gives only a few seconds to a minute warning to reach a toilet. The need to urinate occurs often, including throughout the night, and is also called an *overactive bladder*.
- **Overflow incontinence:** Is the frequent or constant dribbling of urine as a result of the inability to empty the bladder. It never completely empties the bladder and may produce only a weak stream of urine.
- **Mixed incontinence:** Is a combination of symptoms of more than one type of urinary incontinence, such as stress incontinence and urge incontinence.
- **Functional incontinence:** Physical or mental impairment keeps the patient from making it to the toilet in time, such as someone with severe arthritis or Parkinson disease, who may not be able to unbutton his or her pants quickly.
- **Gross total incontinence:** Is the continuous leaking of urine, day and night, or the periodic uncontrollable leaking of large volumes of urine. The bladder has no storage capacity, which is often the result of an anatomic defect.

NURSING IMPLICATIONS

1. Teach the methods of prevention, which include Kegel exercises, frequent trips to the bathroom, wearing a bladder incontinence perineal pad, and the care of a pessary.
2. If surgical intervention is required, provide preoperative and postoperative instructions.
3. Assess for depression, which may result from a decreased quality of life and functional status.

ENDOMETRIOSIS

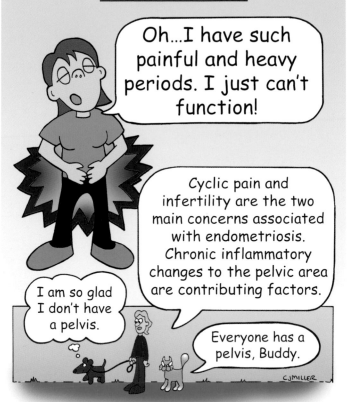

─────── **What You Need to Know** ───────

Endometriosis

DEFINITION

Endometriosis is a condition in which tissue that behaves similar to the cells lining the uterus (endometrium) grows in other areas of the body, causing pain, irregular bleeding, and possible infertility.

SIGNS AND SYMPTOMS

- Pain is the primary symptom, especially painful periods.
- Symptoms
  - Pain in the lower abdomen or pelvic cramps that can be felt for a week or more before menstruation
  - Pain during or after sexual intercourse
  - Pain with bowel movements
  - Pain in the pelvis or low back that may occur at any time during the menstrual cycle
- Other symptoms include fibromyalgia, chronic fatigue syndrome, endocrine disorders, and autoimmune disorders.

MEDICAL MANAGEMENT

- Medications: Nonsteroidal antiinflammatory drugs (NSAIDs) and oral contraceptives
- Surgical intervention: Total abdominal hysterectomy with bilateral salpingo-oophorectomy (TAH-BSO) for women who do not want to have children

NURSING IMPLICATIONS

1. Assess the woman's current understanding of her condition.
2. Provide counseling and education for women about the chronic nature of endometriosis.
3. Refer the woman to support groups.
4. Teach about medication management.
5. Provide preoperative and postoperative teaching if surgical intervention is elected.

Serious/life-threatening implications	Important nursing implications
Common clinical findings	Patient teaching

DYSFUNCTIONAL UTERINE BLEEDING

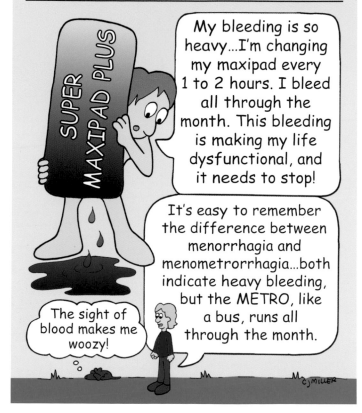

─── **What You Need to Know** ───

Dysfunctional Uterine Bleeding

DEFINITION

Dysfunctional uterine bleeding is excessive uterine bleeding with no demonstrable organic cause—genital or extragenital.

RISK FACTORS

- Anovulation
- Obesity, hyperthyroidism, hypothyroidism, and polycystic ovary syndrome

SIGNS AND SYMPTOMS

- Menstrual periods occur more often than every 21 days or farther apart than 35 days. A normal adult menstrual cycle is 21 to 35 days long. A normal teen cycle is 21 to 45 days.
- Menstrual periods last longer than 7 days. A normal period lasts 4 to 6 days.
- Menses is heavier than normal with the passing of blood clots and soaking through usual pads or tampons each hour for 2 or more hours.
- Profuse bleeding can cause a drop in the hemoglobin (<8 g/dl) and hematocrit (23% to 24%).

MEDICAL MANAGEMENT

- Medications: Oral contraceptives
- Surgical: Dilation and curettage (D&C) and endometrial biopsy

NURSING IMPLICATIONS

1. Assess the woman's current knowledge about the condition.
2. Teach the woman about medications and complications (hemorrhage, passing of blood clots and soaking through usual pads or tampons each hour for 2 or more hours, feeling dizzy) and when to contact a health provider.
3. Provide preoperative and postoperative care if surgery is elected.

Serious/life-threatening implications	Important nursing implications
Common clinical findings	Patient teaching

POLYCYSTIC OVARIAN SYNDROME AND OVARIAN TORSION

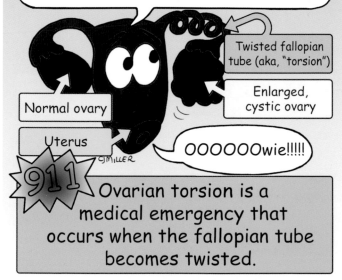

Polycystic ovarian syndrome (PCOS) is an endocrine imbalance that causes ovarian enlargement, cysts, pain, and infertility.

Twisted fallopian tube (aka, "torsion")

Enlarged, cystic ovary

Normal ovary

Uterus

CJMILLER

OOOOOOwie!!!!!

911 Ovarian torsion is a medical emergency that occurs when the fallopian tube becomes twisted.

────── **What You Need to Know** ──────

Polycystic Ovary Syndrome and Ovarian Torsion

DEFINITION

Polycystic ovary syndrome (PCOS) occurs when an endocrine imbalance results in high levels of estrogen, testosterone, and luteinizing hormone (LH) and a decreased secretion of follicle-stimulating hormone (FSH). The ovaries often double in size. *Ovarian torsion* is a twisting of the ovary that compromises blood supply.

RISK FACTORS

- Are associated with problems in the hypothalamic-pituitary-ovarian axis and with androgen-producing tumors
- Can be transmitted as an X-linked dominant or autosomal dominant trait (Stein-Leventhal syndrome)

SIGNS AND SYMPTOMS

- Symptoms include obesity, hirsutism (excessive hair growth), irregular menses or amenorrhea, and infertility.
- Impaired glucose tolerance and hyperinsulinemia may occur; affected women are at high risk for developing type 2 diabetes mellitus and possibly cardiovascular disease.
- Is often diagnosed in adolescence.

MEDICAL MANAGEMENT

- Analgesics may be prescribed for pain management.
- Oral contraceptives (OCs) may be ordered for several months.
- Large cysts (greater than 8 cm) or cysts that do not shrink may be surgically removed (cystectomy).

NURSING IMPLICATIONS

1. Lifestyle modifications (e.g., losing weight) and the management of symptoms such as infertility, irregular menses, and hirsutism are the focus.
2. If pregnancy is not desired, OCs are the usual treatment for irregular menses because they inhibit LH and decrease testosterone levels.
3. Gonadotropin-releasing hormone (GnRH) analogs may be used to treat hirsutism if OCs do not improve this condition. If pregnancy is desired, ovulation-inducing medications are given.
4. Metformin and other insulin medications for type 2 diabetes also are used to lower insulin, testosterone, and glucose levels, which in turn can reduce acne, hirsutism, abdominal obesity, amenorrhea, and other symptoms in women with PCOS.
5. Teaching lifestyle modifications such as exercise and diet may be needed, as well as education about the medications.

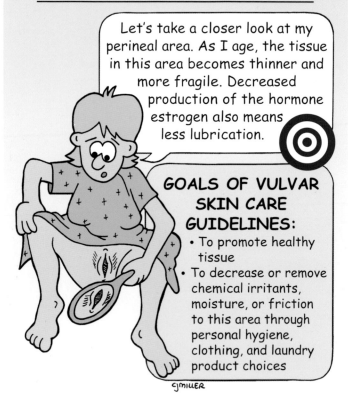

━━━━━━━━━━━━━━━ **What You Need to Know** ━━━━━━━━━━━━━━━

Vulvar Skin Care Guidelines

DEFINITION

Vulvar skin care guidelines promote healthy vulvar skin by decreasing and removing chemicals, moisture, or rubbing (friction).

NURSING IMPLICATIONS

Teach the patient about the following areas to promote vulvar skin care:

Laundry Products
- Use a detergent that is free of dyes and enzymes.
- Do not use fabric softeners or dryer sheets in the washer or dryer.

Clothing
- Wear white, all-cotton underwear, not nylon with a cotton crotch. Cotton allows air in and keeps moisture out. Sleep without underwear or wear loose-fitting cotton boxers or cotton pajama bottoms.
- Avoid wearing panty hose and tight clothing.
- Remove wet bathing and exercise clothing as soon as possible.

Bathing and Hygiene
- Do not use bath soaps, lotions, or gels that contain perfumes.
- Do not use bubble baths, bath salts, or scented oils.
- Do not use soap directly on the vulvar skin.
- Do not apply lotion directly to the vulva.
- Do not scrub vulvar skin with a washcloth. Instead, wash with your hand and warm water; pat dry rather than rubbing with a towel; or use a hair dryer on a cool setting to dry the vulva.
- Use white, unscented toilet paper.
- Do not use feminine hygiene sprays or perfumes or adult or baby wipes. If urine causes burning of the skin, pour lukewarm water over the vulva while urinating. Pat dry rather than wipe.
- Do not use deodorized pads or tampons.
- Do not douche.
- Women may have problems with chronic dampness. Keeping dry is important.
  - Do not wear pads on a daily basis.
  - Choose cotton fabrics whenever possible.
  - Keep an extra pair of underwear and change if dampness is noted.
  - Do not use powders that contain cornstarch.
- Using a lubricant may help dryness and irritation during intercourse.

Birth Control Options
- Lubricated condoms, contraceptive jellies, creams, or sponges may cause itching and burning; avoiding these and using other types of birth control are best.

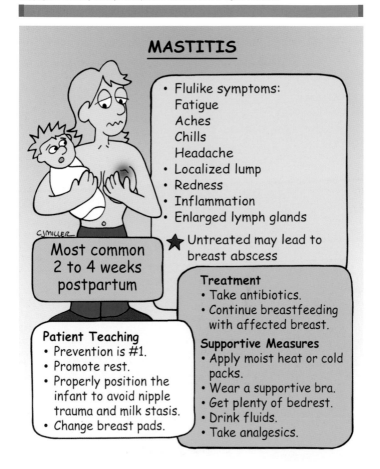

MASTITIS

- Flulike symptoms:
  Fatigue
  Aches
  Chills
  Headache
- Localized lump
- Redness
- Inflammation
- Enlarged lymph glands

★ Untreated may lead to breast abscess

Most common 2 to 4 weeks postpartum

Treatment
- Take antibiotics.
- Continue breastfeeding with affected breast.

Supportive Measures
- Apply moist heat or cold packs.
- Wear a supportive bra.
- Get plenty of bedrest.
- Drink fluids.
- Take analgesics.

Patient Teaching
- Prevention is #1.
- Promote rest.
- Properly position the infant to avoid nipple trauma and milk stasis.
- Change breast pads.

—— **What You Need to Know** ——

Mastitis

DEFINITION

Mastitis is an infection of the breast usually caused by *Staphylococcus aureus*. Mastitis usually occurs in only one breast at time and is often preceded by engorgement or milk stasis in the breast.

RISK FACTORS

- Infection that enters the breast through a damaged nipple, unwashed hands, or the mouth or nose of the infant
- Inadequate emptying of the breasts related to engorgement
- Plugged ducts, abrupt weaning, and a decrease in the number of feedings
- Stress, fatigue, breast trauma, and poor nutrition

SIGNS AND SYMPTOMS

- Usually occurs between weeks 2 and 4 postpartum.
- Flulike symptoms: Chills, fever, headache, and body aches are common.
- Localized warm to hot, reddened area on the breast with tenderness or pain and swelling.
- Infection may have a "pie wedge–shaped" appearance.
- Most commonly occurs in the upper outer quadrant of the breast; may affect one or both breasts.
- Breast abscess is a possible complication.

MEDICAL MANAGEMENT

- Antibiotic (cephalexin or dicloxacillin [10 to 14 days]) therapy or analgesic or antipyretic medications (ibuprofen) are administered.
- Emptying of the breast by breast-feeding or pumping is recommended.

NURSING IMPLICATIONS

1. Promote patient comfort by recommending that she wear a supportive bra and apply warm packs before feeding or pumping.
2. Explain that she should completely empty the breast every 1½ to 2 hours.
3. Promote increased rest, increased fluid intake, and the completion of antibiotic therapy and analgesic and antipyretic medications as needed.
4. Provide encouragement to help the patient sustain her breast-feeding.
5. Teach the patient that the first line of treatment for mastitis is prevention.
6. Teach and reinforce that proper breast-feeding techniques are essential.

Serious/life-threatening implications	Important nursing implications
Common clinical findings	Patient teaching

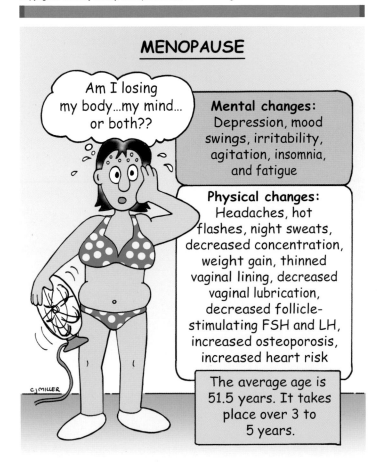

What You Need to Know

Menopause

DEFINITION

Menopause is the complete cessation of menses and occurs when women have not had menstrual flow or spotting for 1 year. *Perimenopause* is the transition period from normal ovulatory cycles to the cessation of menses and is marked by irregular menstrual cycles.

SIGNS AND SYMPTOMS

- Bleeding: Longer periods; 2 to 3 days of spotting, followed by 1 to 2 days of heavy bleeding; or regular menses, followed by 2 to 3 days of spotting
- Genital changes: Low level of estrogen leads to atrophy of vaginal and urethral tissue; membranes become thin, hold less moisture, and lubricate more slowly; increased incidence of vaginitis, dyspareunia
- Urinary frequency, dysuria, uterine prolapse, and stress incontinence
- Hot flush (visible red flush to the skin and perspiration), hot flash (sudden warm sensation in neck, head, and chest), and night sweats (may precipitate sleep deprivation going back to sleep is difficult)
- Mood and behavioral response: Emotionally labile, nervous, agitated, and less control of emotions

MEDICAL MANAGEMENT

- Menopausal hormone therapy: Estrogen replacement or estrogen and progestin replacement; remains highly controversial treatment.

NURSING IMPLICATIONS

1. Provide education about menopause and menopausal hormone replacement.
2. Teach about changes associated with diminishing estrogen levels.
3. Explain physical and emotional changes that occur throughout the perimenopausal period.

| Serious/life-threatening implications | Important nursing implications |
| Common clinical findings | Patient teaching |

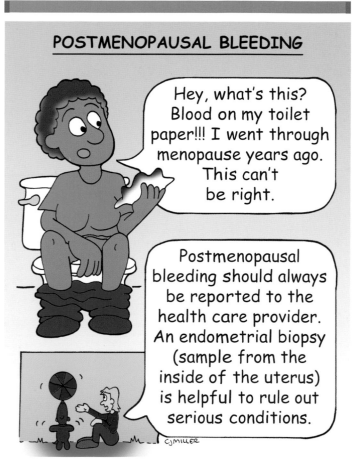

—— **What You Need to Know** ——

Postmenopausal Bleeding

DEFINITION

Postmenopausal bleeding is bleeding after menopause. Even a little spotting is not normal after menopause.

RISK FACTORS

- Polyps: Can develop in the uterus, on the cervix, or inside the cervical canal, and may cause bleeding.
- Endometrial atrophy (thinning of the endometrium): Very thin tissue after menopause, which is caused by diminished estrogen levels, may cause unexpected bleeding.
- Endometrial hyperplasia: May have abnormal cells that can lead to endometrial cancer.
- Hormonal therapy, infection of the uterus or cervix, the use of certain medications, such as anticoagulants, and other types of cancer can cause postmenopausal bleeding.

SIGNS AND SYMPTOMS

- Any vaginal bleeding after the cessation of menses (menopause)

MEDICAL MANAGEMENT

- Transvaginal ultrasound
- Endometrial biopsy
- Hysteroscopy
- Dilation and curettage (D&C)

NURSING IMPLICATIONS

1. Teach the woman to make an appointment to see her health care provider as soon as she has postmenopausal bleeding; it can indicate a number of health problems, some of which are serious.
2. Assess for postmenopausal bleeding in all women who are at risk.

Serious/life-threatening implications	Important nursing implications
Common clinical findings	Patient teaching

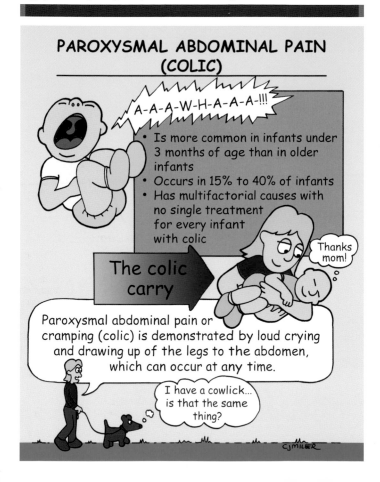

Paroxysmal Abdominal Pain (Colic)

DEFINITION

Paroxysmal abdominal pain or *cramping* (colic) is demonstrated by loud crying and the drawing up of the legs to the abdomen; it can occur at any time. Other definitions relate to the duration of the crying—occurring longer than 3 hours a day, more often than 3 days a week, and longer than 3 weeks, along with parental dissatisfaction with the infant's behavior.

ETIOLOGIC CONSIDERATIONS

- Multifactorial: Too rapid feeding, overeating, swallowing excessive air, and improper feeding technique and position
- Cow's milk allergy (CMA)
- Emotional tension or stress between mother and infant

SIGNS AND SYMTPOMS

- Paroxysmal abdominal pain or cramping, drawing up the legs to the abdomen
- Loud crying
- Self-limiting, generally resolving around 12 to 16 weeks of age

MEDICAL MANAGEMENT

- Sedatives (*Atarax*), antispasmodics, antihistamines, and antiflatulents (*Mylicon*)
- Substitute formula if CMA is suspected.
  - Soy formula is avoided because of a possible sensitivity to soy protein.
  - Hydrolyzed formulas (e.g., Nutramigen, Pregestimil) are extensively used.
  - *Lactobacillus reuteri* is orally administered for colicky, breast-fed infants, along with infants with a mother on a milk-free diet.

NURSING IMPLICATIONS

1. Measures to relieve colic:
   - Place the infant in a prone position over a covered hot-water bottle, heated towel, or covered heating pad.
   - Gently massage the infant's abdomen.
   - "Colic carry" the infant face down with the body across the parent's arm and with the parent's hand under the infant's abdomen while applying gentle pressure.
   - Swaddle the infant.
   - Use bottles that minimize air swallowing; provide smaller and frequent feedings; burp the infant during and after feedings, and place in an upright seat after feeding.
   - If parents smoke, instruct them to smoke outside the house.
2. Reassure and support the parents to prevent trauma as a result of frustration (e.g., shaken baby syndrome).

DIAPER DERMATITIS

Prevention
Is the #1 Goal

- Maintain clean, dry skin.
- Apply zinc oxide to area of developing dermatitis.
- Apply petrolatum (petroleum jelly) barrier to mild dermatitis.
- Identify cause in severe dermatitis with an appropriate intervention.
- Avoid talcum powder.

Nursing Care Management: Alteration of Three Factors

1. Wetness

2. pH

3. Fecal irritants

Diaper Dermatitis

DEFINITION

Diaper dermatitis is an acute inflammatory skin disorder common in infants and either directly or indirectly caused by wearing wet diapers. It is a type of irritant contact dermatitis and may also involve secondary bacterial or yeast infections.

RISK FACTORS

- Prolonged and repetitive contact with an irritant (e.g., urine, feces, soaps, ointments, friction)
- Three principle factors contribute to the development of inflammation: (1) skin wetness, (2) pH of urine, and (3) fecal irritants.

SIGNS AND SYMPTOMS

- Contact irritant: Lesions appear on the convex surfaces or in the skin folds (intertriginous dermatitis) and may have sharply demarcated edges.
- *Candida albicans:* Bright red, confluent lesions with raised borders and satellite lesions are evident.

MEDICAL MANAGEMENT

- Application of zinc oxide or petrolatum (petroleum jelly [Vaseline]) to protect skin
- Topical glucocorticoids (5% to 10%) for resistant inflammation that does not respond to conservative therapy
- Topical antifungals for *Candida albicans* infections

NURSING IMPLICATIONS

1. Prevent diaper dermatitis by keeping the skin dry.
   - Use superabsorbent diapers; change frequently, especially when with stool.
   - If using cloth diapers, use overwraps that allow circulation of air; avoid rubber pants.
2. Apply ointment (e.g., zinc oxide, petrolatum/petroleum jelly) to protect skin.
   - Do not remove protective ointment between changes; remove feces or urine, and reapply.
3. Teach parents to avoid over-washing the skin and using perfumed soaps and commercial disposable wipes.
   - Use mild soap (e.g., Dove).

Serious/life-threatening implications	Important nursing implications
Common clinical findings	Patient teaching

IRON DEFICIENCY ANEMIA

- Irritability
- Tachycardia
- Fatigue
- Glossitis
- Angular stomatitis
- Impaired neurologic and cognitive function
  - ↓ Attention span
  - ↓ Alertness
  - ↓ Learning
- Koilonychia (spoon nails)

Three major causes of disease in children:

(1) Cow's milk as the major food staple for children 12 to 36 months

(2) Rapid growth rate and poor eating habits for adolescents

(3) Preterm infants because related, reduced fetal iron supply

Big Dawg!

Iron Deficiency Anemia

DEFINITION

Iron deficiency anemia is caused by an inadequate supply of dietary iron. Iron stores are usually adequate for the first 5 to 6 months for the term infant (2 to 3 months for the preterm infant); then dietary iron needs to be supplemented to meet growing needs.

RISK FACTORS

- Cow's milk as the major food staple for children from 12 to 36 months
- Rapid growth rate and poor eating habits for adolescents
- Preterm infants, because of reduced fetal iron supply

SIGNS AND SYMPTOMS

- Irritability, tachycardia, fatigue, glossitis, and angular stomatitis are common.
- Neurologic function, such as attention span, alertness, and learning, is impaired.
- Infants may be underweight; however, many are overweight as a result of excess milk ingestion *(milk baby)*.
- Infants may be pale, have poor muscle development, and be prone to infection.

MEDICAL MANAGEMENT

- Diet is managed with iron-fortified formula and cereals (less gastrointestinal symptoms of colic, diarrhea, or constipation).
- Oral iron supplements are usually given for 3 months; vitamin C is administered to facilitate absorption.
  - Given in two divided doses between meals (to aid absorption when the stomach is most free of hydrochloric acid)
  - Do not administer with cow's milk; it interferes with absorption.
- Liquid iron preparation should be taken through a straw to prevent staining the teeth in the older child; teach the child to brush the teeth after taking.
- Z-track for intramuscular (IM) injection of iron dextran is administered.

NURSING IMPLICATIONS

1. Prevent anemia through family education.
2. Administer iron supplement.
3. Teach about diet, and advise the parents that stool may turn to a greenish-black color.
4. Dispel the myth that milk is the "perfect food," especially when it is given to the exclusion of other foods.

CEREBRAL PALSY

- Abnormal muscle tone
  - Decreased sensation

- Decreased communication
  - Decreased cognition

- Decreased coordination
  - Altered mobility

- Seizures
- Hearing and vision impairment

Cerebral palsy is a group of permanent disorders involving the development of movement and posture. It limits activity related to a nonprogressive disturbance in the developing fetal or infant brain.

Cerebral Palsy

DEFINITION

Cerebral palsy (CP) is a group of permanent disorders involving movement and posture. CP limits activity related to a nonprogressive disturbance in the developing fetal or infant brain. Health care practitioners now believe that CP is more often the result of existing prenatal brain abnormalities than it is from birth asphyxia, which has been the prevalent traditional belief in the past.

CLINICAL CLASSIFICATION

- Spastic (pyramidal): Majority of all children with CP
  - Persistent primitive reflexes, positive Babinski sign, exaggerated stretch reflexes, and eventual development of contractures
- Dyskinetic (nonspastic, extrapyramidal)
  - Athetoid (chorea—involuntary, irregular, jerky movements)
  - Dystonic—slow, twisting movements of the trunk or extremities; abnormal posture; difficulties with speech articulation
- Ataxic (nonspastic, extrapyramidal)
  - Wide-based gait; rapid, repetitive movements performed poorly
- Mixed type
  - Combination of spastic and dyskinetic CP

SIGNS AND SYMPTOMS

- Spastic: Hypertonicity, increased deep tendon reflexes (DTRs), scissoring gait, and heel-cord contracture
- Dyskinetic: Purposeless, involuntary, uncontrollable movements of face and extremities, normal DTRs, and rare contracture development
- Ataxic: Disturbed coordination, unsteady gait, and hyporeflexia
- Other: Visual and hearing impairment, drooling, feeding problems, developmental delay, and seizures

NURSING IMPLICATIONS

1. Provide early recognition and promotion of optimal development.
2. Medical therapy is primarily preventative (pain medication, Botox, intrathecal baclofen, antiepileptics) and symptomatic.
3. Promote skills for locomotion, communication, and self-help.
4. Provide educational opportunities to meet the child's needs and capabilities.
5. Promote socialization with other affected and unaffected children.
6. Provide supportive care to the family if orthopedic surgery is required.
7. Teach the family about medications, special feeding methods, physical therapy, and the use of assistive devices (e.g., ankle-foot orthoses [AFOs], wheelchair, braces).

ACUTE GLOMERULONEPHRITIS

- Edema (periorbital and facial)
- Blood pressure (BP)
- Anorexia
- Nausea and vomiting
- Abdominal discomfort
- Dysuria
- Hematuria
- Proteinuria
- Edematous feet

- Headache
- Pallor
- Irritability
- Lethargy

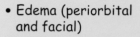

↑ BP

Causes

- Group A β-hemolytic streptococcus (is the most common)
- Pneumococci
- Viral

CJMILLER

Acute Glomerulonephritis

DEFINITION

Acute glomerulonephritis is most commonly a postinfectious disorder caused by group A β-hemolytic streptococcus, pneumococcus, or viral infections. Acute poststreptococcal glomerulonephritis (APSGN) is considered an autoimmune disorder. It is a reaction that occurs as a result of a previous streptococcal infection with certain strains of streptococci and is considered the most common type of acute glomerulonephritis. Most children with APSGN recover completely.

RISK FACTORS

- Streptococcal, pneumococcal, and viral infections

SIGNS AND SYMPTOMS

- Oliguria, edema (periorbital and facial), anorexia, and cola-colored urine
- Pale, irritable, lethargic, and elevated blood pressure
- Older children: Headaches, abdominal discomfort, and dysuria
- Severe cases: Seizures, hypertensive encephalopathy, pulmonary and circulatory congestion, or hematuria in the absence of hypertension and edema

MEDICAL MANAGEMENT

- Antihypertensive drugs: Calcium channel blockers, beta blockers, angiotensin-converting enzyme (ACE) inhibitors
- Diuretics (limited value with severe cases)
- Anticonvulsants for seizures
- Antibiotics for persistent streptococcal infections

NURSING IMPLICATIONS

1. Monitor vital signs, daily body weight, and intake and output (I&O).
2. Bed rest is no longer recommended during the acute phase; ambulation does not have an adverse effect on symptoms or the progression of disease.
3. Encourage frequent rest periods and the avoidance of fatigue.
4. Provide a regular diet with no salt added; sodium is moderately restricted for children with hypertension or edema; protein is restricted for only severe cases of azotemia as a result of prolonged oliguria.
5. Teach parents the importance of follow-up health care.

Serious/life-threatening implications	Important nursing implications
Common clinical findings	Patient teaching

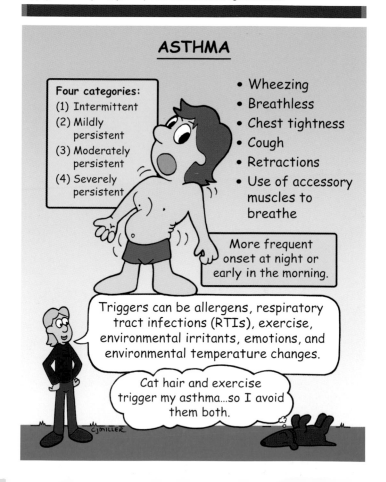

Asthma

DEFINITION

Asthma is a chronic inflammatory disorder of the airways and is considered the most common chronic disease of childhood. The intermittent category has the least number of symptoms with an increase in symptoms or frequency to the last category of severe persistent. The four categories of asthma severity provide a stepwise approach to the medical, environmental, and educational interventions.

RISK FACTORS

- Age, atopy, heredity, and gender (Boys are more affected than girls until adolescence; then the trend reverses.)
- Ethnicity (increased in African Americans), smoking environment

SIGNS AND SYMPTOMS

- Recurrent episodes of wheezing, breathlessness, and chest tightness
- Cough (especially at night and early morning)
- Restlessness, apprehension, and tripod-seated position
- Use of accessory muscles of respiration, barrel chest (repeated episodes), and elevated shoulders

MEDICAL MANAGEMENT

- Conduct pulmonary function tests for diagnosis.
- Peak expiratory flow rate (PEFR): Green, yellow, and red zones; establishing a "personal best value" for each child is needed; this value varies for each child.
- Medications:
  Long-term control medications (preventative): Inhaled corticosteroids, cromolyn sodium, nedocromil, long-acting beta 2–agonists (Serevent), and leukotriene modifiers (Singular)
  Quick-relief medications (rescue): Short-acting beta 2–agonists (albuterol), anticholinergics (Atrovent), and systemic corticosteroids

NURSING IMPLICATIONS

1. Teach the family and child to avoid allergens and known triggers.
2. Relieve bronchospasm; use a peak expiratory flow meter (PEFM) to monitor the condition; administer medications via metered-dose inhaler (MDI).
3. Teach the family how to use an MDI and how to perform controlled breathing exercises.
4. Monitor for status asthmaticus, which is a medical emergency that can result in respiratory failure.

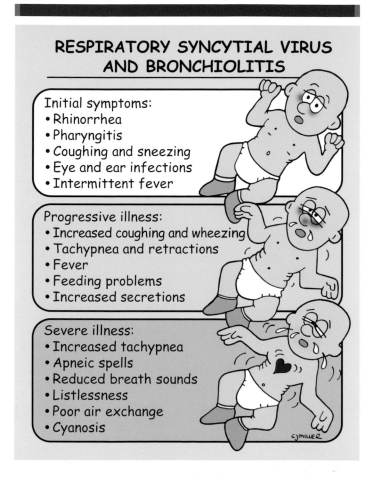

Respiratory Syncytial Virus and Bronchiolitis

DEFINITION

Bronchiolitis is an acute viral infection that occurs primarily in the winter and spring and is most often caused by the respiratory syncytial virus (RSV). Peak incidence of RSV is between 2 and 7 months of age and is transmitted through direct contact with respiratory secretions (e.g., hand to eye, nose, mucous membranes).

RISK FACTORS

- Affects male infants more than female infants; occurs less frequent in breast-fed infants.
- Crowded living conditions increase exposure to respiratory secretions.
- Severe RSV infection in the first year of life increases the risk of developing asthma.

SIGNS AND SYMPTOMS

- Initial: Rhinorrhea, pharyngitis, coughing and sneezing, eye and ear infections, and intermittent fever
- Progressive: Increased coughing and wheezing, tachypnea and retractions, fever, and copious secretions
- Severe: Tachypnea (>70 breaths/min), apneic spells, reduced breath sounds, listlessness, poor air exchange, and cyanosis

MEDICAL MANAGEMENT

- Administer oxygen and intravenous (IV) fluids.

NURSING IMPLICATIONS

1. Maintain contact and standard precautions (i.e., gowns, gloves, meticulous hand hygiene).
2. Monitor oxygen therapy, pulse oximetry, and intravenous (IV) fluids.
3. Frequently assess vital signs (monitor body temperature).
4. Teach breast-feeding mothers to pump and store milk until the infant is stabilized and able to nurse.

Serious/life-threatening implications	Important nursing implications
Common clinical findings	Patient teaching

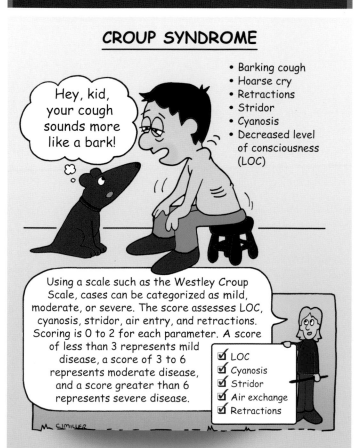

Croup Syndrome

DEFINITION

Croup is a collection of symptoms characterized by hoarseness, barking or brassy cough, and inspiratory stridor resulting from swelling or obstruction of the larynx. Types of croup include acute epiglottis, acute laryngotracheobronchitis, acute spasmodic laryngitis, and acute tracheitis.

ACUTE EPIGLOTTIS

- Is the most serious type, affecting 2- to 5-year-old children; is a rapidly progressive medical emergency.
- Absent or no spontaneous cough, the presence of drooling, and agitation
- High fever, rapid pulse and respirations, and dysphagia

ACUTE LARYNGOTRACHEOBRONCHITIS

- Is the most common type, affecting an infant or child 5 years old and younger. This type is slowly progressive.
- History of upper respiratory infection (URI), inspiratory stridor, suprasternal retractions, barking cough, and hoarseness exists.
- Infants have nasal flaring, intercostal retractions, tachypnea, and continuous stridor.

ACUTE SPASMODIC LARYNGITIS

- Is characterized by paroxysmal attacks of laryngeal obstruction that occur chiefly at night.
- Barking, metallic cough, hoarseness, noisy inspirations, and restlessness are presenting symptoms.
- Child appears anxious and frightened; may have slight hoarseness the next day after the attack.

ACUTE TRACHEITIS

- Occurs in ages 1 month to 6 years and is moderately progressive; is thought to be a complication of laryngotracheobronchitis; however, this type is unresponsive to laryngotracheobronchitis treatment.
- Croupy cough; thick, purulent tracheal secretions; high fever; upper airway obstruction; respiratory failure; and acute respiratory distress syndrome (ARDS) are presenting symptoms.
- May require endotracheal intubation and mechanical ventilation.

Serious/life-threatening implications	Important nursing implications
Common clinical findings	Patient teaching

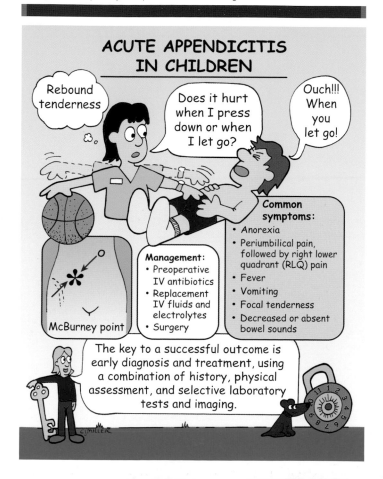

Acute Appendicitis in Children

DEFINITION

Appendicitis is an inflammation of the vermiform appendix—a blind sac at the end of the cecum—that can lead to emergency abdominal surgery during childhood.

RISK FACTORS

- Hardened fecal material (fecalith)
- Swollen lymphoid tissue that often occurs after a viral infection

SIGNS AND SYMPTOMS

- Right left quadrant (RLQ) abdominal pain, fever, rigid abdomen, and decreased or absent bowel sounds
- Vomiting (typically after the onset of pain), nausea, anorexia, referred pain, focal tenderness at McBurney point, and rebound tenderness

MEDICAL MANAGEMENT

- Surgical removal of the appendix; laparoscopic removal for nonperforated cases
- Administration of preoperative intravenous (IV) antibiotics, IV fluids, and electrolytes

NURSING IMPLICATIONS

1. If the patient has severe abdominal pain, do not administer laxatives or enemas; they will stimulate gastrointestinal (GI) motility and increase the risk of perforation.
2. Because children associate the stethoscope with listening, use the bell piece for the initial palpation of the abdomen for tenderness; then provide manual gentle palpation.
3. Allow the child to choose the position most comfortable to him or her, which is usually legs flexed.
4. Administer analgesic medications as ordered.

Serious/life-threatening implications   Important nursing implications

Common clinical findings   Patient teaching

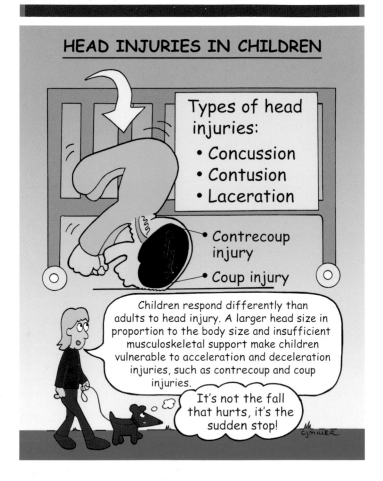

Head Injuries in Children

DEFINITION

A *head injury* is the result of mechanical force or trauma to the scalp, skull, meninges, or brain. Bruising of the brain at the point of impact is the coup injury, and the collision of the brain on the opposite side of the injury is the contrecoup injury; that is, a blow to the occipital region of the brain (coup) can cause injury to the frontal of temporal areas of the brain (contrecoup).

RISK FACTORS

- Falls, motor vehicle accidents, and bicycle injuries

SIGNS AND SYMPTOMS

- Concussion: Alteration in the mental status with or without a loss of consciousness (LOC), confusion, amnesia, fatigue, or headache
- Contusion: Petechial hemorrhages or localized bruising at the coup or contrecoup site of injury; possible focal disturbances in strength, sensation, and visual awareness (i.e., transient weakness of a limb to prolonged unconsciousness and paralysis)
  - Shaken baby syndrome: Profound neurologic impairment, seizures, retinal hemorrhages, and intracranial hemorrhage, along with other skeletal injuries
- Laceration: Penetrating or depressed skull fracture, bleeding around torn brain tissue, and more severe with permanent scarring and some degree of disability

NURSING IMPLICATIONS

1. Monitor for complications—increased intracranial pressure, change in LOC; perform neurologic examinations.
2. Maintain adequate ventilation and bed rest; monitor vital signs.
3. Place the child with the head of the bed slightly elevated and the head in the midline position.
4. Teach the family about long-term rehabilitation of the injured child and preventative strategies for accidents.

Serious/life-threatening implications   Important nursing implications

Common clinical findings   Patient teaching

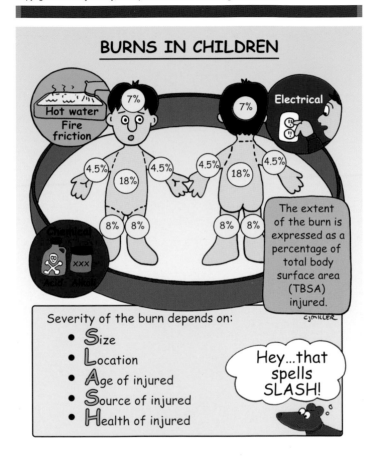

Burns in Children

DEFINITION

A burn injury is categorized as one of three types: thermal, electrical, and chemical. The extent of the burn is expressed as a percentage of total body surface area (TBSA) injured. A modified rule of nines is used for infants and children.

RISK FACTORS

- Home fires, igniting of clothing, playing with matches, and contact with hot surfaces or liquids; maltreatment (nonaccidental injury); sticking objects in electrical outlets, sucking or biting an electrical cord
- Ingesting cleaning or caustic products

SIGNS AND SYMPTOMS: DEPTH OF BURN INJURY

- **Superficial or first-degree burn:** Area is reddened and blanches with pressure; no edema is present; area is generally painful to touch.
- **Partial-thickness or second-degree burn:** Dermis and epidermis are affected; large, thick-walled blisters form; underlying skin is erythematous.
- **Full-thickness or third- and fourth-degree burns:** All of the skin is destroyed; may have damage to the subcutaneous tissue and muscle; usually has a dry appearance, may be white or charred; will require skin grafting to cover the area; underlying structures (e.g., fascia, tendons, bones) are severely damaged, usually blackened.

MEDICAL MANAGEMENT

- Fluid resuscitation; grafting for severe injuries

NURSING IMPLICATIONS

1. Maintain a patent airway and prevent hypoxia.
2. Anticipate the transfer to the burn unit if burns cover more than 15% to 20% of the body surface area.
3. Evaluate fluid status, determine the circulatory status and adequacy of fluid replacement, and obtain child's weight on admission.
   - Assess the status and timeframe of fluid resuscitation; the calculation of fluid replacement begins at the time of the burn injury, not on the arrival at the hospital.
   - Evaluate the renal status and urine output; adequate output for children is 1 ml/kg/hr.
4. Prevent or decrease infection; prevent contractures and scarring.
5. Maintain nutrition and promote positive nitrogen balance for healing.
6. Teach strategies to the family to prevent burn injury.

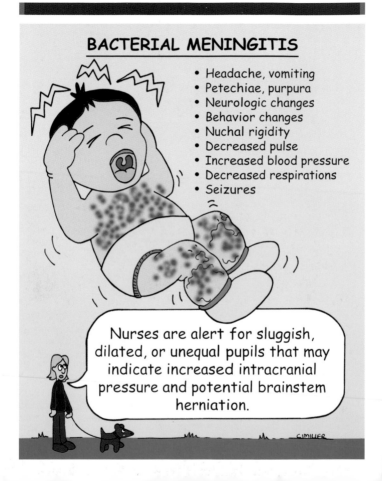

Bacterial Meningitis

DEFINITION

Bacterial meningitis is an acute inflammation of the meningeal tissue covering the brain and spinal cord. The epidemic form is transmitted by droplet infection from nasopharyngeal secretions and occurs predominantly in school-age children and adolescents.

SIGNS AND SYMPTOMS

- Neonates and infants:
  - Fever, bulging fontanel, seizures, and crying with position change
  - Opisthotonos positioning: Dorsal arched position
  - Changes in sleep pattern, increasing irritability, poor sucking; may refuse feedings
  - Poor muscle tone, diminished movement, and irritability
- Children and adolescents:
  - Rash, petechiae, purpura, nuchal rigidity, chills, and high fever
  - Severe and persistent headache, increasing irritability, malaise, changes in level of consciousness, and photophobia
  - Respiratory distress, generalized seizures, nausea, and vomiting
  - Positive Kernig sign: Resistance or pain at the knee and the hamstring muscles when the patient attempts to extend the leg after thigh flexion
  - Positive Brudzinski sign: Reflex flexion of the hips when the neck is flexed

MEDICAL MANAGEMENT

- Isolation precautions, intravenous (IV) antibiotic therapy, IV therapy, and maintenance of ventilation
- Reduction of an increased intracranial pressure (ICP), management of shock, and control of seizures and temperature

NURSING IMPLICATIONS

1. Maintain respiratory isolation precautions.
2. Reduce environmental stimuli with low lights and minimal noise.
3. The side-lying position is the most comfortable for infants because of nuchal rigidity.
4. Take seizure precautions, and monitor for other complications of meningeal irritation.
5. Monitor IV infusions and intake and output (I&O).

Serious/life-threatening implications	Important nursing implications
Common clinical findings	Patient teaching

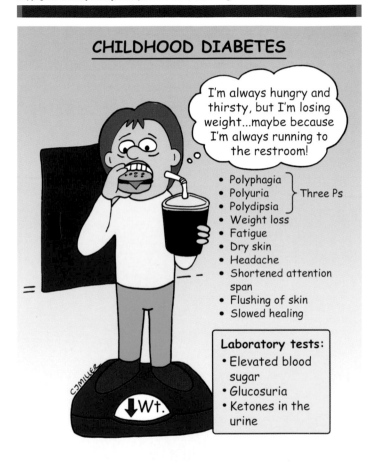

Childhood Diabetes

DEFINITION

Diabetes mellitus is a chronic disorder of metabolism characterized by a partial or complete deficiency of the hormone insulin.

DIAGNOSIS

- Fasting blood glucose above 126 mg/dl; random blood glucose 200 mg/dl accompanied by classic signs of diabetes
- Oral glucose tolerance test (OGTT) finding of 200 mg/dl or more in the 2-hour postprandial sample

SIGNS AND SYMPTOMS

- Polyphagia, polyuria, polydipsia, and abdominal discomfort
- Weight loss, enuresis, irritability, and shortened attention span
- Fatigue, dry skin, poor wound healing, flushed skin, and headache
- Hyperglycemia and diabetic ketoacidosis

MEDICAL MANAGEMENT

- Insulin therapy, diet management, and exercise

NURSING IMPLICATIONS

1. Administer insulin 30 minutes before a meal or snack; do not administer insulin if no carbohydrates are eaten.
2. Maintain adequate fluid intake.
3. Evaluate serum electrolyte levels.
4. Assess the child's current level of knowledge regarding diabetes.
5. Evaluate cultural and socioeconomic parameters.
6. Evaluate child's support system (e.g., family, school).
7. Instruct the child and parents about sick-day guidelines.
8. Promote quality outcomes of blood glucose maintained within normal range, HBA1c range from 6.5% to 8.0%, and prevention of diabetic ketoacidosis.

Serious/life-threatening implications	Important nursing implications
Common clinical findings	Patient teaching

HEMATOLOGIC PROBLEMS—
LEUKEMIA AND HEMOPHILIA

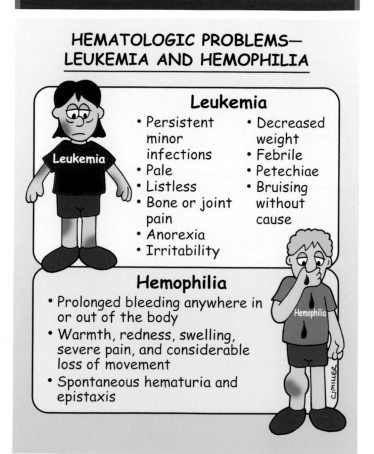

Leukemia

- Persistent minor infections
- Pale
- Listless
- Bone or joint pain
- Anorexia
- Irritability
- Decreased weight
- Febrile
- Petechiae
- Bruising without cause

Hemophilia

- Prolonged bleeding anywhere in or out of the body
- Warmth, redness, swelling, severe pain, and considerable loss of movement
- Spontaneous hematuria and epistaxis

Hematologic Problems—Leukemia and Hemophilia

LEUKEMIA

Leukemia is an uncontrolled proliferation of abnormal white blood cells. Eventual cellular destruction occurs as a result of the infiltration of the leukemic cells into the body tissue.

- Three primary consequences of leukemia: (1) anemia from red blood cell (RBC) destruction and bleeding; (2) infection associated with neutropenia; and (3) bleeding tendencies caused by decreased platelets
- Two forms of leukemia: Acute lymphocytic leukemia (ALL), (blast or stem cell), which is the most common form, and acute myelogenous leukemia (AML)
- Symptoms of leukemia: Fever, pallor, fatigue, anorexia, hemorrhage (petechiae), bone and joint pain, and vague abdominal pain

Nursing Intervention

- Centers around the therapy: Myelosuppression, drug toxicity, and leukemic infiltration cause secondary complications that require supportive care.
- Prepare family for diagnostic and therapeutic procedures.
- Provide continual emotional support that corresponds to treatment phases:
  - Induction: Complete remission or clinical disappearance of symptoms
  - Intensification or consolidation: Decreases the total tumor burden
  - Maintenance: Further chemotherapy to ensure remission

HEMOPHILIA

Hemophilia is a defect in the clotting mechanism. Classically, there are two types, distinguishable only by laboratory tests. The disease is most often recognized during the toddler stage. Clinically, the two types are the same, but both may occur in varying degrees of severity.

  Hemophilia A: factor VIII deficiency (classic hemophilia)
  Hemophilia B: factor IX deficiency (Christmas disease)

Symptoms

- Persistent or prolonged bleeding: Occurs from minor trauma or insults, hemarthrosis (bleeding into joint cavities), spontaneous hematuria, or hematoma.
- Intracranial hemorrhage: May be fatal.
- Petechiae: Are uncommon because platelet count is normal.

Nursing Intervention

- Teach family the early recognition of signs and symptoms of hemophilia for those with a genetic history.
- Prevent bleeding, and recognize and control bleeding episodes.
- Treat bleeding episodes with factor replacement.
- Prevent crippling effects of bleeding (e.g., hemarthrosis).
- Promote an exercise program; teach home care management to the parents.